Clinical Pharmacy and Therapeutics

Clinical Pharmacy and Therapeutics

Basavaraj K Nanjwade M Pharm, PhD
Professor
Department of Pharmaceutics
KLE University's College of Pharmacy
Belgaum, Karnataka, India

Jigar M Patel M Pharm
Department of Pharmaceutics
KLE University's College of Pharmacy
Belgaum, Karnataka, India

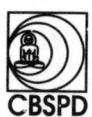

CBS Publishers & Distributors Pvt Ltd

New Delhi • Bengaluru • Chennai • Kochi • Kolkata • Lucknow • Mumbai
Hyderabad • Jharkhand • Nagpur • Patna • Pune • Uttarakhand

Clinical Pharmacy and Therapeutics

ISBN: 978-93-87085-17-6

©Publisher

First Edition: 2011

CBS Reprint: 2018, 2019, 2023, **2025**

Published by **Satish Kumar Jain** and produced by **Varun Jain** for

CBS Publishers & Distributors Pvt Ltd
4819/XI Prahlad Street, 24 Ansari Road, Daryaganj, New Delhi 110 002, India.
Ph: 011-23266838, 23289259   Website: www.cbspd.com
                                  e-mail: delhi@cbspd.com

Corporate Office: 204 FIE, Industrial Area, Patparganj, Delhi 110 092
Ph: 011-4934 4934   Fax: 011-4934 4935
                                e-mail: publishing@cbspd.com; publicity@cbspd.com

Branches

* **Bengaluru:** Seema House 2975 17th Cross, KR Road, Banasankari 2nd Stage, Bengaluru 560 070, Karnataka, India
  Ph: +91-80-26771678/79   Fax: +91-80-26771680   e-mail: bangalore@cbspd.com
* **Chennai:** 7, Subbaraya Street, Shenoy Nagar, Chennai 600 030, Tamil Nadu, India
  Ph: +91-44-26680620, 26681266   Fax: +91-44-42032115   e-mail: chennai@cbspd.com
* **Kochi:** 42/1325, 1326, Power House Road, Opp KSEB, Power House, Ernakulum Kochi 682 018, Kerala, India
  Ph: +91-484-4059061-65,67   Fax: +91-484-4059065   e-mail: kochi@cbspd.com
* **Kolkata:** 147, Hind Ceramics Compound, 1st Floor, Nilgunj Road, Belghoria, Kolkata-700056, West Bengal, India
  Ph: +033-25633055, 033-25633056   e-mail: kolkata@cbspd.com
* **Lucknow:** Basement, Khushnuma Complex, 7 Meerabai Marg (Behind Jawahar Bhawan), Lucknow-226001, UP, India
  Ph: +0522-4000032   e-mail: tiwari.lucknow@cbspd.com
* **Mumbai:** PWD Shed, Gala no 25/26, Ramchandra Bhatt Marg, Next to JJ Hospital Gate no. 2, Opp. Union Bank of Inc
  Noorbaug, Mumbai-400009, Maharashtra, India
  Ph: 022-66661880/89   e-mail: mumbai@cbspd.com

Representatives

* **Hyderabad**   0-9885175004   * Jharkhand   0-9811541605   * Nagpur   0-8692091830
* Patna   0-9334159340   * Pune   0-9664372571   * Uttarakhand   0-9716462459

Printed at Chaman Enterprises, Daryaganj, Delhi, India

PREFACE

Clinical pharmacy and therapeutics involves brief introduction to clinical pharmacy, basic concepts of pharmacotherapy, important disorders of organ systems and their management, and concept of essential drugs and rational drug use. This book explains detail study of important disorders and concept of pharmacotherapy.

This book describes major disorders such as cardiovascular diseases, CNS disorders, respiratory disorders, gastro intestinal diseases, endocrine disorders, infectious diseases etc. This book also describes clinical pharmacokinetics and individualization of drug therapy, adverse drug reaction, drug interaction, interpretation of the clinical laboratory tests in the basic concepts of pharmacotherapy. Concept of essential drugs and the rational drug usage is also mentioned in this book.

The objective of writing this book is to present this subject in a simple way and make it as informative as possible. Although this book is targeted to the undergraduate and postgraduate students, it caters to anyone who is interested or working in the R&D department of an industry, clinician, and research scholars.

Although, several books of foreign authors are available in the market, in most of books not all the chapters are covered in a single book or they are not simple enough to follow from the student's point of view. Very few books are available from the Indian authors. The growing importance of this subject and my love for this wonderful subject has inspired me to write this book. I hope to inspire students and other readers through this book to understand and appreciate the application of clinical pharmacy and therapeutics in various pharmaceutical field such as product development, R&D, hospitals etc.

The authors express their sincere thanks and appreciation to Prof. Dr. F. V. Manvi Principal and Prof. Ashok D. Taranalli Vice Principal, KLE University College of Pharmacy, Belgaum. Also to Prof. Dr. Chandrakant K. Kokate Vice-Chancellor and Prof. Dr. P. F. Kotur Registrar, KLE University, Belgaum, Karnataka, India for rendering useful suggestions and inputs, apart from being intensely persuasive to complete the project.

We are grateful to Mr. Gowrishetty Madhusudhan IKON BOOKS publication who has taken keen interest and spared no pains for the fine getup of book.

Authors

Table of Contents

Part C Neoplastic diseases

Chapter 7 Therapeutic Drug Monitoring(TDM)

Chapter 8 Concept of Essential and Rational drug use

Chapter 1

INTRODUCTION TO CLINICAL PHARMACY

1.1 INTRODUCTION

Now adays many countries face problems in delivering health care because of less awareness, improper guidance, and technologies but that must be recognized by the pharmacists if the profession of pharmacy is to flourish. In doing so, one cannot help but recognize the opportunities for professional practice. There are various branches of pharmacy which are primarily concerned with manufacturing, procurement, preparation, distribution and control of drug products. The concept of patient oriented approach in addition to the traditional product oriented approach has clearly emerged out. The term clinical pharmacy is being used to describe this new role of the pharmacists which comprises functions necessary to discharge a particular set of social responsibilities related to therapeutic drug use in the following major categories:

1. Prescribing drugs

2. Dispensing and administering drugs

3. Documenting professional services

4. Reviewing drug use

5. Education

6. Direct patient involvement

7. Consultation

In short clinical pharmacy is control on drug use and the effective application of health knowledge, skills and ethics that assures optimal safety in the distribution and use of medicine. Clinical pharmacy includes involvement in prescribing rounds, patient counseling, drug history taking, monitoring for adverse drug reaction and interaction. There are several minor activities conducted are Health education, Training and education of own staff and doctor's and nurses, clinical trials, case references, Research and clinical meetings. Clinical pharmacy has bought the pharmacist into closer touch with the prescribers and details of treatment of patients.

Clinical Pharmacy may be defined as "The active participation of hospital pharmacists in patient care with the long term aim of giving advice on medication with an individual patient in mind and tailoring drug therapy for that individual."

"Profession of Clinical Pharmacy will advance only through the primary goals of quality patient care".

"Clinical pharmacy is a concept or philosophy emphasizing the safe and appropriate use of drugs in patients. It places the emphasis of drugs on the patient not on the product. It is achieved only by interacting responsible for drugs with health disciplines which are in any way concerned with drugs."

1.2 AIM OF CLINICAL PHARMACY

The aim of clinical pharmacy is to ensure the patient's maximum well-being and to play a meaningful role in safe and rational use of the drugs. The main goals of the clinical pharmacy are:

- To assist the physician in doing a better job of prescribing and monitoring drug therapy for patient.

- To assist medical and para-medical staff and documenting medication incidents correctly.

- To maximise the patient's compliance in drug use process.

1.3 BASIC COMPONENTS OF THE CLINICAL PHARMACY

There are some basic components of the clinical role in the practice of pharmacy are:

1. **Communication Skill:** The clinical pharmacist should have good communication skill, in order to communicate with the patient and co-professionals freely and effectively.

2. **Clinical Skill:** The clinical pharmacist should have thorough knowledge about etiology of a disease, signs, symptoms, pathophysiology, laboratory tests, pharmacokinetics, etc. He should be clinically trained for providing information on rational drug use, related drug therapy and for reviewing drug doses.

3. **Professional Relationship:** He should be able to understand and appreciate the role of medical and para-medical staff wherever possible. He must accompany physician on medical rounds to assist him by providing drug information. The physician, pharmacist and nurses should develop an inter-professional relationship with each other to enhance the quality of patient care.

4. **Empathy:** Clinical pharmacist should possess a deep sense of shared responsibility towards medical care of patients. It will help him in tacking medication history and gaining patient's confidence.

5. **Monitoring Drug Therapy:** Clinical pharmacist must help in monitoring drug therapy because it is an on-going process and keeps on changing depending upon patient's conditions.

1.4 OBJECTIVES OF CLINICAL PHARMACY

The primary objective of clinical pharmacy is to improve pharmaceutical services and increase health care delivery services to the patient and to the paramedical and medical professionals in the community and the institutions. There must be close collaboration between the university faculties, community practitioners, institutional practitioners, pharmacy students and professional associations for objectives of the clinical pharmacy.

Pharmacy education has a vital role in establishing objectives for clinical pharmacy. The American Association of College of Pharmacy

(AACP) has adopted the following objectives for instruction in clinical pharmacy.

1. To help, make the student more aware of the general methods of diagnosis and patient care specifically as they related to drug therapy.

2. To develop in the student a facility for effective interaction with the patient and with practitioners of other health professions.

3. To help the student, develop a patient awareness in providing pharmaceutical services.

4. To acquaint the student with clinical application of pharmacological and pharmaceutical principles.

5. To enable the student to integrate the knowledge acquired in the preclinical years and apply it to the solution of the real problems.

6. To develop in the student an awareness of his responsibility in monitoring drug utilization.

The other important objectives in relation to community practitioners, institutional practitioners and professional associations are as follows;

1. To optimize the individual drug therapy by maximizing drug effectiveness and minimizing the adverse drug effects.

2. To assist the physicians in doing a better job of prescribing and monitoring drug therapy.

3. To assist the nurses in administering medications and documenting medication incidents correctly.

4. To maximize the patients role in the drug use process.

1.5 SCOPE OF CLINICAL PHARMACY

Clinical pharmacy services are of considerable importance in all the hospitals because clinical pharmacist serves as a guide to physician for safe and rational use of the drugs. A clinical pharmacist can help to achieve economy in the hospital by planning safe drug policies, suggesting means of reductions of waste, by preventing misuse or pilferage of drug and in the preparation of budget by forecasting the future drug need of hospital, based upon their drug utilization patterns. Hence scope of the clinical pharmacy is of almost appreciation in following areas:

1. Drug Information

The provision of drug information is the foundation of clinical pharmacy practice. The pharmacist must realize the importance of literature and utilize the information retrieval techniques to make data available in a rapid efficient manner. The drug information centers can be tremendous resource and which serves as data bank of important information. The drug information not only provided by verbal discussion but also provided via an intrahospital news letter, in-service education and community lectures.

2. Drug Utilization

The pharmacist has a professional obligation to monitor drug utilization. He should be ever mindful about (1) Drug abuse (2) Abnormal prescribing patterns (3) Drug – Drug interactions (4) Drug – food interactions (5) drug – laboratory test interactions.

3. Drug Distribution

The pharmacist must have complete understanding and appreciation of the various drug distribution systems are essential for communication with other health professionals and public regarding unit-dose packaging, unit-dose systems of distribution and control procedures.

4. Drug Evaluation and Selection

The pharmacist becomes a valuable resource person in the selection of drugs for various diseases states and he can provide unique services in evaluating the formulation of various dosage forms. Pharmacists with knowledge of Biopharmaceutics and the ability to apply this knowledge for the patients benefit can provide a unique service in drug evaluation and selection.

5. Pharmacy Education and Teaching

The pharmacists have fundamental knowledge and expertise that should be shared with all those involved in drug storage, preparation, prescribing and administration.

1.6 ROLE OF CLINICAL PHARMACY SERVICES

1. Supervise all drug distribution activities for drug use control and patient safety.

2. Selects for patients therapeutically effective prescription drug products at reasonable cost.

3. Records patients medication history of drugs taken and any adverse reactions therefrom.

4. Detects and diagnoses adverse drug reactions and drug interactions.

5. Counsels patients on the use of the drugs to assure compliance.

6. Advises patients on selection of OTC drugs.

7. Helps to establish dosage regimens for patients.

8. Promotes rational drug therapy by physicians.

9. Integrates the psycho-socio-economic aspects of health care.

10. Supervises management of patients with acute and chronic diseases.

11. Detects and overcomes incompatibilities in drug mixtures.

12. Compounds drug preparations to meet specific patient requirement.

13. Supervises the dispensing of prescriptions by dispensing assistants.

14. Has ability to evaluate the drug literature.

15. Performs drug utilization review.

16. Provides health care education to the public.

17. Prescribes for mild self limiting diseases.

18. Monitors patients responses to drugs utilizing patient medication profile and other resources.

The following diagram illustrates the role of clinical pharmacist in various areas of making decisions nondrug therapy.

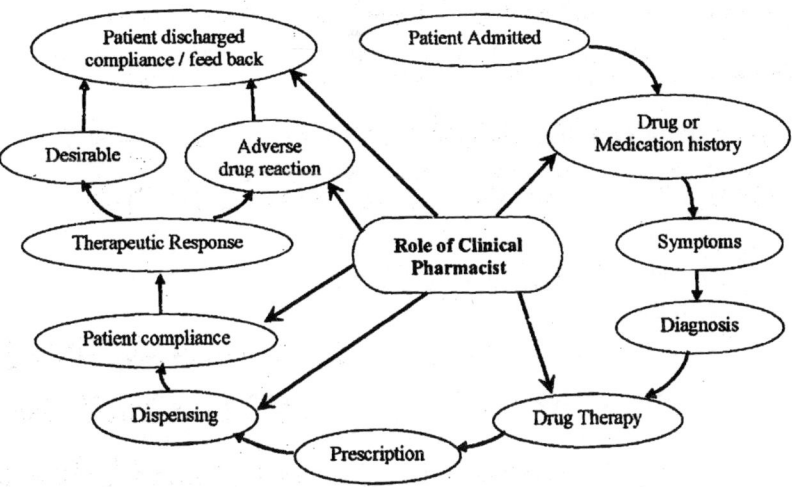

Fig. 1: Schematic Role of a Clinical Pharmacist

- **Taking medication history of the patient:** Clinical pharmacist must take and maintain the history of patient by interacting with him. He should document the hyper sensitivities or allergy to certain drugs, food habbits, drug dependence or intoxications with chemicals, side effects of some drugs, incorrect drug administration, etc. This will help in saving physician's efforts and will result in faster and more accurate therapy.

- **Drug Interactions:** Many OTC drugs have potential to interact with prescription drugs. After receiving the prescription, pharmacist checks the drug interaction and patient's habits with the help of patients history record.

- **Selection of proper drug therapy:** Clinical pharmacist can assist in selection of a proper drug product/generic formulation, depending on the considerations of bio-availability and bio-equivalence of such products.

- **Adverse drug Reactions:** Patients with hepatic disorders or kidney impairment are more prone to adverse drug reactions. Patients having more than one pathological complaint with multiple drug therapy generally face such problems. Clinical pharmacist can help is detection, prevention and reporting of adverse drug reactions. He can suggest physician for alternate therapy wherever necessary.

- **Drug Informations:** Clinical Pharmacist has the knowledge and expertise to provide detailed information on medicines to members of health profession and the public. He can abstract the information from periodic bulletins or news letters and provide the same to physician on matter pertaining to pharmacokinetics and dynamics of drugs.

Finally clinical pharmacy, is that area within the pharmacy curriculum which deals with patient care with emphasis on drug therapy. Clinical pharmacist participates in patient education programmes, drug use profiles, research and development programmes of the hospital etc., apart from many other activities. It ensures the appropriate and safe use if the drug in patient cure.

REVIEW QUESTIONS

ESSAY QUESTIONS

1. Write a short notes on the concept of Clinical Pharmacy .
2. Write briefly about computer applications in Clinical Pharmacy.
3. Enumerate the qualities of a Clinical Pharmacist.
4. Discuss the role of Clinical Pharmacist in health care team.
5. Write about the history of Clinical Pharmacy.
6. Describe Medicines Management Cycle.

SHORT ANSWER QUESTIONS

1. Explain different sources of errors.
2. Enumerate the aims of Pharmaceutical care.
3. Write a short note on Drug therapy assessment.
4. Describe the role of Clinical Pharmacy in reducing the risks.
5. What is the Discipline of Clinical Pharmacy?

Chapter *2*

BASIC CONCEPTS OF PHARMACOTHERAPY

2.1 INTRODUCTION

The goal of pharmacotherapy is to provide optimal drug therapy in the treatment or prevention of disease. This goal can be achieved with larger variability in pharmacological effect which observed with drug administration. The important intervening steps or processes, which occur following drug dosing that lead to therapeutic effects both beneficial and toxic in the body, as describe in fig. 1 which show the dose effect relationship.

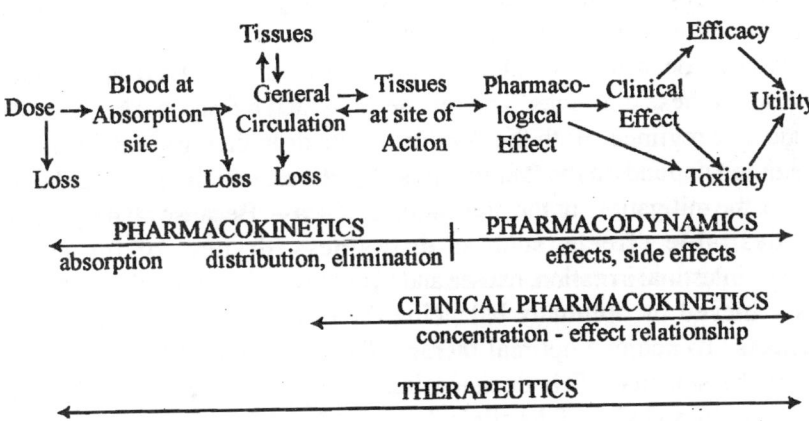

Fig. 1. Schematic representation of the dose-effect relationship for a drug.

2.2   CLINICAL PHARMACOKINETICS

"Pharmacokinetics is the study of kinetics of absorption, distribution, metabolism and excretion (ADME) of drugs and their corresponding pharmacologic, therapeutic, or toxic responses in man and animals." Applications of pharmacokinetics studies include:

- Bioavailability measurements

- Effects of physiological and pathological conditions on drug disposition and absorption

- Dosage adjustment of drugs in disease states, if and when necessary

- Correlation of pharmacological responses with administered doses

- Evaluation of drug interactions

- **Clinical prediction:** using pharmacokinetic parameters to individualize the drug dosing regimen and thus provide the most effective drug therapy.

Those patients who suffer from chronic ailments such as diabetes and epilepsy may have to take drugs every day for the rest of their lives. At the other extreme are those who take a single dose of a drug to relieve an occasional headache. The duration of drug therapy is usually between these extremes. The manner in which a drug is taken is called a dosage regimen. Both the duration of the drug therapy and the dosage regimen depend on the therapeutics objectives, which may be either the cure, the mitigation, or the prevention of disease. Because all drug exhibit undesirable effects, such as drowsiness, dryness of the mouth, gastrointestinal irritation, nausea and hypotension, successful drug therapy is achieved by optimally balancing the desirable and the undesirable effects. To achieve optimal therapy, the appropriate "drug of choice" must be selected. This decision implies an accurate diagnosis of the disease, knowledge of the clinical state of the patient. Then the questions How much? How often? And How long? must be answered. The question How much? recognizes that the magnitudes of the therapeutics and toxic responses are functions of the dose given. The question How often?

recognizes the importance of time, in that the magnitude of the effect eventually declines with time following a single dose of the drug. The question How long? recognizes that a cost (in terms of side effect, toxicity, and economics) is incurred with continuous drug administration. In practice, these questions cannot be divorced from one another. For example, the convenience of giving a larger dose less frequently may be more than offset by an increased incidence of toxicity.

During the drug development process, large numbers of patients are tested to determine optimum dosing regimens, which are then recommended by the manufacturer to produce the desired pharmacologic response in the majority of the anticipated patient population. However, intra- and interindividual variations will frequently result in either a sub therapeutic (drug concentration below the MEC) or toxic response (drug concentrations above the minimum toxic concentration, MTC), which may then require adjustment to the dosing regimen. Clinical pharmacokinetics is the application of pharmacokinetic methods to drug therapy. Clinical pharmacokinetics involves a multidisciplinary approach to individually optimized dosing strategies based on the patient's disease state and patient-specific considerations.

Table 1. Ratio of Age-Adjusted Death Rates, by Male/Female Ratio from the 10 Leading Causes of Death in the USA, 2003

Disease	Rank	Male: Female
Disease of heart	1	1.5
Malignant neoplasms	2	1.5
Cerebrovascular diseases	3	4.0
Chronic lower respiration diseases	4	1.4
Accidents and others*	5	2.2
Diabetes mellitus	6	1.2
Pneumonia and influenza	7	1.4
Alzheimers	8	0.8
Nephrotis, nephrotic syndrome and nephrosis	9	1.5
Septicemia	10	1.2

The study of clinical pharmacokinetics of drugs in disease states requires input from medical and pharmaceutical research which is a list of 10 age-adjusted rates of death from 10 leading causes of death in the United States, 2003. The influence of many diseases on drug disposition is not adequately studied. Age, gender, genetic, and ethnic differences can also result in pharmacokinetic differences that may affect the outcome of drug therapy. The study of pharmacokinetic differences of drugs in various population groups is termed as population Pharmacokinetics.

Pharmacokinetics is also applied to therapeutic drug monitoring (TDM) for very potent drugs such as those with a narrow therapeutic range, in order to optimize efficacy and to prevent any adverse toxicity. For these drugs, it is necessary to monitor the patient, either by monitoring plasma drug concentrations (e.g., theophylline) or by monitoring a specific pharmacodynamic endpoint such as prothrombin clotting time (e.g., warfarin). Pharmacokinetic and drug analysis services necessary for safe drug monitoring are generally provided by the clinical pharmacokinetic service (CPKS). Some drugs frequently monitored are the amino glycosides and anticonvulsants. Other drugs closely monitored are those used in cancer chemotherapy, in order to minimize adverse side effects.

2.3 INDIVIDUALIZATION OF DRUG THERAPY

The goal of clinical pharmacokinetics or pharmacodynamic is to develop individualized drug therapy regimens to maximize the likelihood of therapeutic success. The doses utilized in clinical practice typically are derived from phase II/III clinical trials in which the safety and efficacy of an agent are evaluated. The information from clinical trials as well as preclinical work from animal and in-vitro studies provides data on the doses necessary to obtain concentrations in the "usual therapeutic range." As discussed previously, the therapeutics range defines the range of concentrations in which most patients have therapeutic effect and a low incidence of toxicity; however for drugs exhibiting a narrow therapeutics index, it may be necessary to more precisely define the dosage regimen for an individual based on (1) patient factors (severity of disease), (2) concentrations achievable at site of drug action (distribution, elimination) and (3) the level of sensitivity to the drug (Pharmacodynamics),

Not all drugs require rigid individualization of the dosage regimen. Many drugs have a large margin of safety (i.e. exhibit a wide therapeutic window), and strict individualization of the dose is unnecessary. The U.S. Food and Drug Administration (FDA) have approved an *over-the-counter* (OTC) classification for drugs that the public may buy without prescription. In the past few years, many prescription drugs, such as ibuprofen, loratidine, omeprazole, naproxen, nicotine patches, and others, have been approved by the FDA for OTC status. These OTC drugs and certain prescription drugs, when taken as directed, are generally safe and effective for the labeled indications without medical supervision. For drugs that are relatively safe and have a broad safety-dose range, such as the penicillins, cephalosporins, and tetracyclines, the antibiotic dosage is not dose titrated precisely but is based rather on the clinical judgment of the physician to maintain an effective plasma antibiotic concentration above a minimum inhibitory concentration.

For drugs with a narrow therapeutic window, such as digoxin, aminoglycosides, antiarrhythmics, anticonvulsants, and some antiasthmatics, such as theophylline, individualization of the dosage regimen is very important. The objective of the dosage regimen design for these drugs is to produce a safe plasma drug concentration that does not exceed the minimum toxic concentration or fall below a critical minimum drug concentration below which the drug is not effective. For this reason, the dose of these drugs is carefully individualized to avoid plasma drug concentration fluctuations due to intersubject variation in drug absorption, distribution, or elimination processes. For drugs such as phenytoin that follow nonlinear pharmacokinetics at therapeutic plasma drug concentrations, a small change in the dose may cause a huge increase in the therapeutic response, leading to possible adverse effects.

The monitoring of plasma drug concentrations is valuable only if a relationship exists between the plasma drug concentration and the desired clinical effect or between the plasma drug concentration and an adverse effect. For those drugs in which plasma drug concentration and clinical effect are not related, other pharmacodynamic parameters may be monitored. For example, clotting time may be measured directly in patients on warfarin anticoagulant therapy. For asthmatic patients, the bronchodilator, albuterol, is given by inhalation via a metered-dose inhaler and the patient's FEV_1 (forced expiratory volume) may be used as a measure of drug efficacy. In cancer chemotherapy, dose adjustment for individual patients may depend on the severity of side effects and the patient's ability to tolerate the drug. For some drugs that have large inter- and intrasubject variability, clinical judgment and experience with the drug is needed to dose the patient properly.

2.4 SPECIAL PRECAUTIONS IN DRUG USAGE DURING INFANCY AND IN THE ELDERLY (PEDIATRICS & GERIATRICS).

Our smallest family members are also our most vulnerable to accidents in the home. Because of their lack of knowledge and experience, and their natural inquisitiveness, kids want to explore everything - even things that are dangerous. By taking a few simple steps, we can greatly reduce the dangers they face. When babies are first born, they're totally helpless. You'll need to take extra precautions with infants, and while some of these safety tips may seem obvious to you, there are others that may not be so obvious.

One way to promote a good outcome when administering drug therapy is to call on your knowledge of normal growth and development in children and your knowledge of safe administration techniques for specific route.

Oral Route:

- Drug volume should not exceed that which can be swallowed by a very small mouth. The drug dose should be mixed in small amount of liquid so the entire dose is taken.

- Avoid adding a drug dose to formula. The infant may refuse future feeding because of the foul taste.

- Balance dosage schedules with feeding schedules. Consider whether the drug should be given with meals or on an empty stomach. Check for possibilities of food drug interaction.

IM Route:

- Assess whether a less painful route is possible.

- If the IM route is unavoidable, apply a topical, local anesthetic, such as lidocaine and prilocaine combination (EMLA cream), to numb the injection site.

- Locate anatomic landmarks and boundaries of injection sites.

- Evaluate muscle mass, skin condition, and potential complications related to the child's diagnosis.

- Seek help to hold the child still while administering the IM injection.

- In infants, neither the deltoid nor the dorsogluteal muscles site is used because muscles masses are too small and undeveloped. The ventrogluteal muscle site, which is large at birth, is not recommended for use in infants because problems encountered in positioning the child make it difficult to locate the muscle site accurately.

IV Route:

- Minimize initial pain in starting the IV by applying topical anesthetic.

- Check the IV inserter site hourly for infiltration in infants and children.

- Monitor fluid status for signs of over load (risk is greatest in neonates and young infants because their immature kidney function).

- Supply no more then 1 hour's worth of fluid when administering a continuous IV drip with an infusion pump (in case the pump manifunction).

- Drug may be administered IV to the infants through peripheral site. Ideally select site that is easy to access and that poses the least risk to the patients. In infants and neonate, the scalp's many superficial veins offer easy access.

Table 2 summarizes the changes that occur with aging and the possible pharmacokinetic effect in the elderly patients.

Table 2. Factors Altering Drug Response in the Elderly

Age-Related Changes	Effect on Drug Therapy
Decrease gastric acidity, decreased gastric motility	Possible decrease or delayed absorption
Dry mouth and decreased saliva	Difficulty swallowing oral drugs
Decreased liver blood flow, decreased liver mass	Delayed and decreased metabolism of certain drugs, possible increased effect, leading to toxicity
Decreased lipid content of content of the skin	Possible decrease in absorption of transdermal drugs
Increased body fat, decreased body water	Possible increase in toxicity of water-soluble drugs, more prolonged effects of fat-soluble drugs
Decreased serum proteins	Possible increased effect and toxicity of highly protein-bound drugs
Decreased renal mass, blood flow, and glomerular filtration rate	Possible increased serum levels, leading to toxicity of drugs excreted by the kidney
Changes in sensitivity of certain drug receptors	Increase or decrease in drug effect

2.5 DRUG USAGE IN PREGNANCY AND LACTATION

Objectives

- To discuss the reasons for avoiding, or minimizing drug therapy during pregnancy and lactation.

- Describe the selected teratogenic drugs.

- Outline the guideline for drug therapy of pregnancy-associated signs and symptoms.

- Discuss the guideline for drug therapy of selected chronic disorders during pregnancy and lactation.

- Discuss the safety to immunization given during pregnancy.

- Teach women to avoid prescribed and over the counter drug when possible and to inform physicians and dentists if there is a possibility of pregnancy.

- Discuss the role of the home care nurse working with the pregnant women.

- Discuss the drug use during pregnancy complication (e.g. preterm labour, preeclampsia, selected infections) and normal labour and delivery in terms of their effects on the mother and newborn infant.

Introduction

Drug use before and during pregnancy and during lactation require special consideration and, in general, should be avoided or minimized when possible, in sexually active women of reproductive age and ability who may become pregnant, the concern is that the women may ingest drugs that are potentially harmful to the fetus before she knows she is pregnant.

The use of any medication-prescription or nonprescription-carries a risk of causing birth defects in the developing fetus. Drugs administered to pregnant women, particularly during the first trimester (3 months), may cause teratogenic effects. A **teratogen** is any substance that causes abnormal development of the fetus leading to a severely deformed fetus. Drugs are one type of teratogen. In an effort to prevent teratogenic effects, the FDA has established five categories suggesting the potential of a drug for causing birth defects (Fig. 3). Information regarding the pregnancy category of a specific drug is found in reliable drug literature, such as the inserts accompanying drugs and approved drug references. In general, most drugs are contraindicated during pregnancy or lactation unless the potential benefits of taking the drug outweigh the risks to the fetus or the infant.

During pregnancy, no woman should consider taking any drug, legal or illegal, prescription or nonprescription, unless the drug is prescribed or recommended by the primary health care provider. Smoking or drinking any type of alcoholic beverage also carries risks, such as low birth weight, premature birth, and fetal alcohol syndrome. Children born of mothers using addictive drugs, such as cocaine or heroin, often are born with an addiction to the drug abused by the mother.

Pregnancy – Associated Symptoms and Their Management

Anemia

Three types of anemia are common during pregnancy.

I.   Physiologic anemia

II.   Iron-deficiency anemia

III.   Megaloblastic anemia

Physiologic anemia, which results from expanded blood volume. Iron-deficiency anemia, which is related to long term nutritional deficiencies. Iron supplements are usually given for prophylaxis and I should be taken with the food to decrease gastric irritation.

Constipation

Constipation often occurs during pregnancy, if laxative required, a bulk producing agent (e.g. Metamucil; Benefibre) is the most physiologic for the mother and safest for the fetus because it is not absorbed systemically. A stool softener or an occasional saline laxative may also be used. Mineral oil should be avoided because it interferes with absorption of fat-soluble vitamins.

Nausea and Vomiting

Nausea and vomiting often occurs, especially during early pregnancy. Dietary management and maintaining fluid and electrolyte balance are recommended. Anti-emetic drugs should be given only if nausea and vomiting are severe enough to threaten the mother's nutritional or metabolic status.

Pregnancy Categories A
• Controlled studies show no risk to the foetus
• Adequate well-controlled studies in pregnant women have not demonstrated risk to the foetus

Pregnancy Categories B
• There is no evidence of risk in humans
• Animal studies show risk, but human findings do not
• If no adequate human studies have been done, animal studies are negative

Pregnancy Categories C
• Risk cannot be ruled out
• Human studies are lacking, and animal studies are either positive for foetal risk lacking
• The drug may be used during pregnancy if the potential benefits of the drug outweigh its possible risks

Pregnancy Categories D
• There is positive evidence of risk to the human foetus
• Investigational or postmarketing data show risk to the foetus.
• However, potential benefits may outweigh the risk to the foetus. If needed in a life-threatening situation or a serious disease, the drug may be acceptable if safer drugs cannot be used or are ineffective

Pregnancy Categories X
• Use of the drug is contraindicated in pregnancy
• Studies in animals or humans or investigational or postmarketing reports, have shown foetal risk that clearly outweighs any possible benefit to the patient.

Regardless of the pregnany category or the presumed sfatey of the drug, no drug should be administered during pregnancy unless it is clearly needed and the potential benefits outweigh harm to the foetus.

Fig. 2. Pregnancy Categories

Pregnancy-induced Hypertension

Pregnancy-induced hypertension includes preeclampsia and eclampsia, conditions that endanger the lives of mother and fetus. Preeclampsia is most likely to occur during the third trimester of pregnancy, before, during and after delivery. It is manifested by hypertension and proteinuria.

2.6 DRUG REACTIONS

Drugs produce many reactions in the body. The following sections discuss adverse drug reactions, allergic drug reactions, drug idiosyncrasy, drug tolerance, cumulative drug effect, and toxic reactions. Pharmacogenetic reactions can also occur. A pharmacogenetic reaction is a genetically determined adverse reaction to a drug.

Adverse Drug Reactions

Patients may experience one or more **adverse reactions** (side effects) when they are given a drug. Adverse reactions are undesirable drug effects. Adverse reactions may be common or may occur infrequently. They may be mild, severe, or life threatening. They may occur after the first dose, after several doses, or even after many doses. An adverse reaction often is unpredictable, although some drugs are known to cause certain adverse reactions in many patients. For example, drugs used in the treatment of cancer are very toxic and are known to produce adverse reactions in many patients receiving them. Other drugs produce adverse reactions in fewer patients. Some adverse reaction is predictable, but many adverse drug reactions occur without warning.

Some texts use both terms *side effect* and *adverse reactions.* These texts distinguish between the two terms by using *side effects* to explain mild, common, and nontoxic reactions; *adverse reaction* is used to describe more severe and life-threatening reactions. For the purposes of this text only the term *adverse reaction* is used, with the understanding that these reactions may be mild, severe, or life threatening.

Allergic Drug Reactions

An **allergic reaction** also is called a **hypersensitivity** reaction. Allergy to a drug usually begins to occur after more than one dose of the drug is given. On occasion, the nurse may observe an allergic reaction the first time a drug is given because the patient has received or taken the drug in the past.

A drug allergy occurs because the individual's immune system views the drug as a foreign substance or **antigen.** The presence of an antigen stimulates the antigen-antibody response that in turn prompts the body to produce **antibodies.** If the patient takes the drug after the antigen–antibody response has occurred, an allergic reaction results.

Even a mild allergic reaction produces serious effects if it goes unnoticed and the drug is given again. Any indication of an allergic reaction is reported to the primary health care provider before the next dose of the drug is given. Serious allergic reactions require contacting the primary health care provider immediately because emergency treatment may be necessary.

Some allergic reactions occur within minutes (even seconds) after the drug is given; others may be delayed for hours or days. Allergic reactions that occur immediately often are the most serious. Allergic reactions are manifested by a variety of signs and symptoms observed by the nurse or reported by the patient. Examples of some allergic symptoms include itching, various types of skin rashes, and hives (urticaria). Other symptoms include difficulty breathing, wheezing, cyanosis, a sudden loss of consciousness, and swelling of the eyes, lips, or tongue.

Anaphylactic shock is an extremely serious allergic drug reaction that usually occurs shortly after the administration of a drug to which the individual is sensitive. This type of allergic reaction requires immediate medical attention. Symptoms of anaphylactic shock are listed in Fig. 4.

All or only some of these symptoms may be present. Anaphylactic shock can be fatal if the symptoms are not identified and treated immediately. Treatment is to raise the blood pressure, improve breathing, restore cardiac function, and treat other symptoms as they occur. Epinephrine (adrenalin) 0.1 to 0.5 mg may be given by subcutaneous or intramuscular injection. Hypotension and shock may be treated with fluids and vasopressors. Bronchodilators are given to relax the smooth muscles of the bronchial tubes. Antihistamines may be given to block the effects of histamine.

Table 4. Symptoms of Anaphylactic Shock

Respiratory	Bronchospasm
	Dyspnea (difficult breathing
	Feeling of fullness in the throat
	cough
	Wheezing
Cardiovascular	Extremely low blood pressure
	Tachycardia (heart rate > 100 bpm)
	Palpations
	Syncope (fainting)
	Cardiac arrest
Integumentary	Urticaria
	Angioedema
	Pruritis (itching)
	Sweating
Gastrointestinal	Nausea
	Vomiting
	Abdominal pain

Angioedema (angioneurotic edema) is another type of allergic drug reaction. It is manifested by the collection of fluid in subcutaneous tissues. Areas that are most commonly affected are the eyelids, lips, mouth, and throat, although other areas also may be affected. Angioedema can be dangerous when the mouth is affected because the swelling may block the airway and asphyxia may occur. Difficulty in breathing or swelling to any area of the body is reported immediately to the primary health care provider.

Toxic Reactions

Most drugs can produce **toxic** or harmful reactions if administered in large dosages or when blood concentration levels exceed the therapeutic level. Toxic levels build up when a drug is administered in dosages that exceed the normal level or if the patient's kidneys are not functioning properly and cannot excrete the drug. Some toxic effects are immediately visible; others may not be seen for weeks or months. Some drugs, such as lithium or digoxin, have a narrow margin of safety, even when given in recommended dosages. It is important to monitor these drugs closely to avoid toxicity.

Drug toxicity can be reversible or irreversible, depending on the organs involved. Damage to the liver may be reversible because liver cells can regenerate. However, hearing loss due to damage to the eighth cranial nerve caused by toxic reaction to the anti-infective streptomycin may be permanent. Sometimes drug toxicity can be reversed by the administration of another drug that acts as an antidote. For example, in serious instances of digitalis toxicity, the drug Digibind may be given to counteract the effect of digoxin toxicity.

Nurses must carefully monitor the patient's blood levels of drugs to ensure that they remain within the therapeutic range. Any deviation should be reported to the primary health care provider. Because some drugs can cause toxic reactions even in recommended doses, the nurse should be aware of the signs and symptoms of toxicity of commonly prescribed drugs.

Pharmacogenetic Reactions

A **pharmacogenetic disorder** is a genetically determined abnormal response to normal doses of a drug. This abnormal response occurs because of inherited traits that cause abnormal metabolism of drugs. For example, individuals with glucose-6-phosphate dehydrogenase (G6PD) deficiency have abnormal reactions to a number of drugs. These patients exhibit varying degrees of hemolysis (destruction of red blood cells) if these drugs are administered. More than 100 million people are affected by this disorder. Examples of drugs that cause hemolysis in patients with a G6PD deficiency include aspirin, chloramphenicol, and the sulfonamides.

2.7 DRUG INTERACTIONS

It is important for the nurse administering medications to be aware of the various drug interactions that can occur, most importantly drug–drug interactions and drug–food interactions. The following section gives a brief overview of drug interactions. Specific drug–drug and drug–food interactions are discussed in subsequent chapters.

Drug-Drug Interactions

A drug-drug interaction occurs when one drug interacts with or interferes with the action of another drug. For example, taking an antacid with oral tetracycline causes a decrease in the effectiveness of the tetracycline. The antacid chemically interacts with the tetracycline and impairs its absorption into the bloodstream, thus reducing the effectiveness of the tetracycline. Drugs known to cause interactions include oral anticoagulants, oral hypoglycemics, anti-infectives, antiarrhythmics, cardiac glycosides, and alcohol. Drug-drug interactions can produce effects that are additive, synergistic, or antagonistic.

- *Additive Drug Reaction:* An additive drug reaction occurs when the combined effect of two drugs is equal to the sum of each drug given alone. For example, taking the drug heparin with alcohol will increase bleeding. The equation one + one = two is sometimes used to illustrate the additive effect of drugs.

- *Synergistic Drug Reaction:* Drug synergism occurs when drugs interact with each other and produce an effect that is greater than the sum of their separate actions. The equation one + one = four may be used to illustrate synergism. An example of drug synergism is when a person takes both a hypnotic and alcohol. When alcohol is taken simultaneously or shortly before or after the hypnotic is taken, the action of the hypnotic increases. The individual experiences a drug effect that is greater than if either drug was taken alone. On occasion, the occurrence of a synergistic drug effect is serious and even fatal.

- *Antagonistic Drug Reaction:* An antagonistic drug reaction occurs when one drug interferes with the action of another, causing neutralization or a decrease in the effect of one drug. For example, protamine sulfate is a heparin antagonist. This means that the administration of protamine sulfate completely neutralizes the effects of heparin in the body.

Drug-Food Interactions

· When a drug is given orally, food may impair or enhance its absorption. A drug taken on an empty stomach is absorbed into the bloodstream at a faster rate than when the drug is taken with food in the stomach. Some drugs (e.g., Captopril) must be taken on an empty stomach to achieve an optimal effect. Drugs that should be taken on an empty stomach are administered 1 hour before or 2 hours after meals. Other drugs, especially drugs that irritate the stomach, result in nausea or vomiting, or cause epigastric distress, are best given with food or meals. This minimizes gastric irritation. The nonsteroidal anti-inflammatory drugs and salicylates are examples of drugs that are given with food to decrease epigastric distress. Still other drugs combine with a drug forming an insoluble food-drug mixture. For example, when tetracycline is administered with dairy products, a drug-food mixture is formed that is unabsorbable by the body. When a drug is unabsorbable by the body, no pharmacologic effect occurs.

2.8 INTERPRETATION OF CLINICAL LABORATORY TESTS

A key to taking control of your health is learning to monitor your immune system. The bulk of immune monitoring is done through a variety of blood tests. Learning how to read and understand your laboratory tests can be quite frustrating. This article will provide basic information to help with this process. Because different labs reports results a little differently, it may be wise to ask your doctor to help you read the results as well.

There are some basic rules which hold true for nearly all laboratory tests:

1.   Different laboratories can get different results from the same

sample of blood. Make sure you ask your doctor which lab as used if it was noted on the report.

2. Laboratories can make mistakes. If your results have changes dramatically since your last test, have it run again.

3. Most lab values have to be interpreted along with other clinical and laboratory data in order to develop a meaningful diagnosis. Very seldom will only one value give all of the answers.

4. Laboratory values differ according to age, sex, current medications, etc. Therefore, the interpretation of these values needs to be done with these parameters in mind.

5. The 'normal' range is the value that is normal for a person who does not have HIV infection. For example, a low cholesterol value in an HIV positive individual is not uncommon.

Complete Blood Count (CBC)

The complete blood count (CBC) is one of the most common tests offered by a doctor. It is a routine test used to evaluate the blood and general health. Asymptomatic, HIV positive people should have this test done twice a year. Symptomatic people should have their CBC done at least every three months. Additionally, if you are on anti-HIV medication you might have to have this test more often. A CBC measures all of the following parameters: red blood cell count (RBC), white blood cell count (WBC), hemoglobin, hematocrit, three red cell indices, and the white cell differential. Platelet cunts are sometimes included in a CBC.

Red Blood Cell Count (RBC)

The RBC count is the number of red blood cells in a cubic millimeter of blood. The RBCs are the cells produced in the bone marrow that carry oxygen to your tissues. The normal rage is $4.5 - 5.9$ million/ mm^3 for men and 4.0 - 5.3 million/mm^3 for women. A slightly decreased value is not cause for alarm as many individuals with HIV have values below the normal range. However, a markedly decreased value should be thoroughly investigated. A person with significant low RBC count can have symptoms of fatigue, shortness of breath, and appear pale in colour. A low RBC count can be due to progressive HIV illness or to certain medications or both. AZT, for example, can suppress the production of RBCs in some people. A decrease in the RBC count usually causes a decrease in the hemoglobin and hematocrit values.

White Blood Cell Count (WBC)

The WBC count is the number of white blood cells in a cubic centimeter of blood. The primary function of these cells is to prevent and fight infections. There are many different types of white blood cells that play specific roles in fighting infections. These specific types of WBCs can be measured in a white cell differential. Normal WBC count is from 4,500 to 11,000. The WBC count can be decreased for a variety of reasons: certain medications decrease their production in the bone marrow, minor viral infections which you may not even be aware of, stress, and opportunistic infections can all change WBC counts. Values markedly decrease should be cause for concern, since during this situation one is more susceptible to other infections.

Hemoglobin

Oxygen is carried to the tissues via hemoglobin in the red blood cells. A normal hemoglobin level is 14 - 18 g/dl for men and 12 - 16 g/dl for women. A slow progressive decline in hemoglobin is often seen in people with AIDS. This is usually due to a decline in the number of RBCs produced in the bone marrow. Any drug which causes a suppression of the bone marrow will decrease the hemoglobin levels. In most cases it's a matter of balancing the effects of the drug with it's potential side effects. When the side effects become too great, either the drug must be discontinued or the dose reduced to a tolerable level. A drug which mimics the action of the hormone erythropoietin (a.k.a. Procrit, EPO and newer brand names), has it's effect on the bone marrow causing the production of new RBCs. It has provided great relief to thousands of individuals of people with HIV and kidney dialysis patients. EPO has enabled many people to stay on bone marrow suppressive drugs without the need for transfusions.

Hematocrit

The hematocrit is the percent of the cellular components in your blood to the fluid or blood plasma. This test is one of the truest markers of anemia. Normal values for men are 40-54% ad for women, 37-47%. A decrease in hematocrit is always seen with a decrease in hemoglobin. These two values are linked to one another.

Mean Cell Volume (MCV)

The mean cell volume or MCV is the most important of the RBC indices. It is a measure of the average size of the RBC. For those individuals taking AZT the MCV will always be normally elevated, i.e. greater than 100. Vitamin B12 and Folic Acid deficiency also causes increases in MCV. Normal MCV levels are 80 - 96.

Platelets

Platelets are cellular fragments which are necessary for the blood to clot. When activated by trauma, platelets migrate to the site of injury where they become 'sticky' - adhering to the injured site and helping to form a fibrin clot or scab. Normal platelet values are 150,000 - 450,000. In some individuals, HIV itself causes a decrease in the number of platelets. Otherwise, drugs can also cause low platelet counts. Even though counts are considered low below 150,000, most people can survive without the threat of internal bleeding with counts above 50,000. On very rare occasions, the numbers of platelets present are adequate, but for unknown reasons they don't function correctly. Any malady involving one's platelets can be a potentially serious condition.

White Cell Differential

The white cell differential counts 100 white cells and differentiates them by type. This gives a percent of the different kinds of white cells in relation to one another. The three main types are: polymorphonuclear cells (PMNs), lymphocytes, and monocytes. PMNs are increased during bacteria infections, while lymphocytes are decreased with viral infections. Increased monocytes are sometimes seen in chronic infections. Normal percent of PMNs is 55 - 80%. 25 - 45% is the normal number of lymphocytes, and 2 - 10% is normal for monocytes.

There are wide ranges of blood chemistry tests which are done on individuals either routinely or for specific reasons. Some of the ones pertaining to HIV are mentioned below.

Cholesterol

Cholesterol levels, as mentioned earlier, are routinely decreased in HIV positive individuals. It's not understood why this occurs, but it is thought to be related to altered metabolism. Normal cholesterol levels are 150 - 250 mg/dl.

Amylase

Amylase is an enzyme that is secreted in the mouth by the salivary glands and also in the pancreas. It can be an early warning sign of acute pancreatitis when elevated. ddI can cause problems with the pancreas in a small number of people taking the drug. Normal amylase levels are 25 - 125 milliunits/ml.

CPK or CK

CPK or CK is an enzyme that's found in the brain and muscles of the body. Strenuous exercise as well as heart attack can cause increases in CPK. This makes clear the point of elevating an abnormal test result in the context of other factors. Myopathy, dysfunction/distress with the muscles, can sometimes be confirmed with an elevated CPK. Myopathy is usually caused by HIV but can also b due to AZT, especially at higher dosages. Normal levels of this enzyme are 1 - 80 milliunits/ml (30 degrees 0 or 55 - 170 milliunits/ml (37 degrees). Values will be slightly lower for women.

Liver Function Tests

Liver function tests include 5 - 6 individual tests which collectively can help determine the status of ones liver. Elevated liver enzymes are most often caused by certain medications. The HIV positive population also has a high prevalence of hepatitis. At least 4 different viruses are known to cause hepatitis, all leading to increased liver function tests. Therefore, compound factors can be at work. If liver enzymes are only moderately elevated, most doctors will take a 'wait and see' attitude, monitoring them over a period of a few weeks to a few months. However, if elevation is quite high, the underlying factor must be found. This might very well be one of the medications that you are currently taking. The names of these liver function tests include SGOT, SGPT, alkaline phos, total bilirubin, and LDH.

Kidney Function Tests

Two tests which measure kidney function are the BUN and Creatinine. The usefulness of these two tests in an HIV positive individual usually relates to medications possibly toxic o the kidneys. Hence kidney function is monitored in this way. Foscarnet is an example of a drug which can cause renal toxicity. Normal BUN levels are 10 - 20 mg/dl. Normal levels of Creatinine are 0.6 - 1.1 mg/dl.

Lymphocyte Subsets

The category of lymphocyte subsets includes absolute counts and percentages of CD4 and CD8 cells as well as other parameters. Usually the number and percent of B cells is included and the number and percent of all lymphocytes (except those called 'natural killer' or NK cells). Lymphocytes are broken down mainly into CD4 (+) cell and CD8 (+) cells. It is well known that HIV causes a slow progressive decline in the number and percent of CD4 (+) cells in most individuals. There are exceptions. Some people progress in their disease rapidly and others don't seem to progress much at all after more than 12 or 13 years. Normal CD4 counts are 350 - 1500. The role of CD8 cells is less clearly understood. Early on in the epidemic, high CD8 cell counts caused inversion of the CD4:CD8 ratio and was thought to adversely affect illness. Now it is generally believed that elevated CD8 counts are advantageous since its thought to keep HIV somewhat constrained. Normal CD8 cell counts in an HIV negative person is 275 - 780.

REVIEW QUESTIONS

ESSAY QUESTIONS

1. Write notes on forms of Patient counselling.

2. Explain the concepts of NDDS and their therapeutic usefullness with examples.

3. a. Explain the terms ' Bioavailability' and ' Bioequivalence'.

    b. How will you find out the Bioavailability of a drug following oral administration of controlled release systems.

4. Write short notes on a) Invivo Drug Interactions
   b) Renal clearance of drugs in infants.

5. What are the factors influencing the hepatic metabolism of drugs?

6. What are various pharmacokinetic and pharmacodynamic parameters that are to be considered in designing drug delivery system.

7. a.Write a note on Monteux test and Vidal test and their clinical significance.

   b.How will you use the data pertaining to serum creatinine and serum urea nitrogen levels to assess the functioning of kidneys?

8. Write a brief note on ELISA test and its significance.

9. Describe in detail with respect to drug drug interactions with examples.

10. Briefly explain about different clinical lab tests.

11. Write short notes on the following:

    a.Factors to be considered for fixing dosagre regimen for long term therapy.

    b.Iatrogenic diseases.

    c.Clinical significance of Glucose tolerance test.

SHORT ANSWER QUESTIONS

1. Write a note on individualisation of drug therapy.

2. Write a note on drug interactions giving different classification with suitable examples.

3. Write short notes on following terms with their importance in clinical pharmacokinetics.

   a.Area Under Curve   b. t½

4. Give Short notes on Iatrogenic diseases and Drug delivery systems.

5. Explain Briefly about Clinical toxicology.

6.   Enumerate Adverse drug reactions.

7.   Write about pharmaco economic analytical methods.

8.   Discuss about Type A adverse drug reactions.

9.   Write short notes on Clinical significance of serum creatinine and bilirubin.

Chapter 3

DISORDERS OF ORGAN SYSTEMS AND THEIR MANAGEMENT

PART A CARDIOVASCULAR DISORDERS

3.1 HYPERTENSION

Blood pressure is the force of the blood against the walls of the arteries. Blood pressure rises and falls throughout the day. When the blood pressure stays elevated over time, hypertension develops. A systolic pressure less than 120 mm Hg and a diastolic blood pressure of less than 80 mm Hg (120/80) are considered optimal. **Hypertension** is usually defined as a systolic pressure above 140 mm Hg and a diastolic pressure above 90 mm Hg. Table 1 identifies blood pressure levels for adults and implications of diagnosis. Patients in the high-normal range require frequent blood pressure monitoring; patients in stage 1, 2, or 3 should be under the care of a physician. Hypertension is serious because it causes the heart to work too hard and contributes to atherosclerosis. It increases the risk of heart disease, congestive heart failure, kidney disease, blindness, and stroke.

Table 1. Blood Pressure Levels for Adults

CATEGORY	SYSTOLIC(in mm Hg)		DIASTOLIC(in mm Hg)
Optimal	Less than 120	and	Less than 80
Normal	Less than 130	and	Less than 85
High-normal	130-139	and	85-89
HYPERTENSION			
Stage 1	140-159	or	90-99
Stage 2	160-179	or	100-109
Stage 3	180 or higher	or	110 or Higher

Most cases of hypertension have no known cause. When there is no known cause of hypertension, the term **essential hypertension** is used. Essential hypertension has been linked to certain risk factors, such as diet and lifestyle. Following are the risk factors which, associated with hypertension.

- Smoking

- Age (women older than 65 years and men older than 55 years of age)

- Obesity

- Diabetes

- Lack of physical activity

- Chronic alcohol consumption

- Family history of cardiovascular disease

- Sex (men and postmenopausal women)

In the United States, African-Americans are twice as likely as Caucasians to experience hypertension. After age 65 years, African-American women have the highest incidence of hypertension. Essential hypertension cannot be cured but can be controlled. Many individuals experience hypertension as they grow older, but hypertension is not a part of healthy aging. For many older individuals, the systolic pressure gives the most accurate diagnosis of hypertension.

Once essential hypertension develops, management of this disorder becomes a lifetime task. When a direct cause of the hypertension can be identified, the condition is described as **secondary hypertension.** Among the known causes of secondary hypertension, kidney disease ranks first, with tumors or other abnormalities of the adrenal glands following. In **malignant hypertension** the diastolic pressure usually exceeds 130 mm Hg. In secondary hypertension, taking care of the medical condition causing the hypertension results in the patient regaining a normal blood pressure.

Malignant hypertension is a dangerous condition that develops rapidly and requires immediate medical attention. Patients with malignant hypertension experience organ damage as the result of hypertension. Target organs of hypertension include the heart, kidney, and eyes (retinopathy).

Most primary care providers will prescribe lifestyle changes to reduce risk factors before prescribing drugs. The primary care provider may recommend measures, such as weight loss (if the patient is overweight), reduction of stress, regular aerobic exercise, quitting moking (if applicable), and dietary changes, such as a decrease in sodium (salt) intake. Most people with hypertension are "salt sensitive," that is that any salt or sodium more than the minimal bodily need is too much for them and leads to an increase in blood pressure. Dietitians usually recommend the Dietary Approaches to Stop Hypertension (DASH) diet. Studies indicate that blood pressure was reduced by eating a diet low in saturated fat, total fat, and cholesterol and rich in fruits, vegetables, and low-fat dairy foods. The DASH diet includes whole grains, poultry, fish, and nuts and has reduced amounts of fats, red meats, sweets and sugared beverages. The diet is rich in potassium, calcium, magnesium, protein, and fiber. Stress-reducing techniques, such as relaxation techniques, meditation, and yoga, may also be a part of the treatment regimen.

When drug therapy is begun, the primary care provider may first prescribe a diuretic or beta (β) blocker because these drugs have been shown to be highly effective. However, as in many other diseases and conditions, there is no "best" single drug, drug combination, or medical regimen for treatment of hypertension. After examination and evaluation of the patient, the primary care provider selects the antihypertensive drug and therapeutic regimen that will probably be most effective.

The types of drugs used for the treatment of hypertension include:

- Vasodilating drugs for example, hydralazine (Apresoline) and minoxidil (Loniten).

- β-adrenergic blocking drugs for example, Atenolol (Tenormin), metoprolol (Lopressor), and propranolol (Inderal).

- Antiadrenergic drugs (centrally acting) for example, guanabenz (Wytensin) and guanfacine (Tenex).

- Antiadrenergic drugs (peripherally acting) for example, guanadrel (Hylorel) and guanethidine (Ismelin).

- Alpha (α)-adrenergic blocking drugs for example, doxazosin (Cardura) and prazosin (Minipress).

- Calcium channel blocking drugs for example, amlodipine (Norvasc) and diltiazem (Cardizem).

- Angiotensin-converting enzyme (ACE) inhibitors for example, captopril (Capoten), enalapril (Vasotec), and lisinopril (Prinivil).

- Angiotensin II receptor antagonists for example, irbesartan (Avapro), losartan (Cozaar), and valsartan (Diovan).

- Diuretics for example, furosemide (Lasix) and hydrochlorothiazide (HydroDIURIL).

Mechanism of action

Many antihypertensive drugs lower the blood pressure by dilating or increasing the size of the arterial blood vessels **(vasodilatation)**. Vasodilatation creates an increase in the **lumen** (the space or opening within an artery) of the arterial blood vessels, which in turn increases the amount of space available for the blood to circulate. Because blood volume (the amount of blood) remains relatively constant, an increase in the space in which the blood circulates (i.e. the blood vessels) lowers the pressure of the fluid (measured as blood pressure) in the blood vessels. Although the method by which antihypertensive drugs dilate blood vessels varies, the result remains basically the same. Antihypertensive drugs that have vasodilating activity include:

- Adrenergic blocking drugs

- Antiadrenergic blocking drugs

- Calcium channel blocking drugs

- Vasodilating drugs

Another type of antihypertensive drug is the diuretic. The mechanism by which the diuretics reduce elevated blood pressure is unknown, but it is thought to be based, in part, on their ability to increase the excretion of sodium from the body.

The mechanism of action of the ACE inhibitors is not fully understood. It is believed that these drugs may prevent (or inhibit) the activity of **Angiotensin-converting enzyme,** which converts Angiotensin I to Angiotensin II, a powerful vasoconstrictor. Both angiotensin I and ACE normally are manufactured by the body and are called **endogenous** substances. The vasoconstricting activity of angiotensin II stimulates the secretion of the endogenous hormone aldosterone by the adrenal cortex. **Aldosterone** promotes the retention of sodium and water, which may contribute to a rise in blood pressure. By preventing the conversion of angiotensin I to angiotensin II, this chain of events is interrupted, sodium and water are not retained, and the blood pressure decreases. The angiotensin II receptor antagonists act to block the vasoconstrictor and aldosterone effects of angiotensin II at various receptor sites, resulting in a lowering of the blood pressure (Fig. 1).

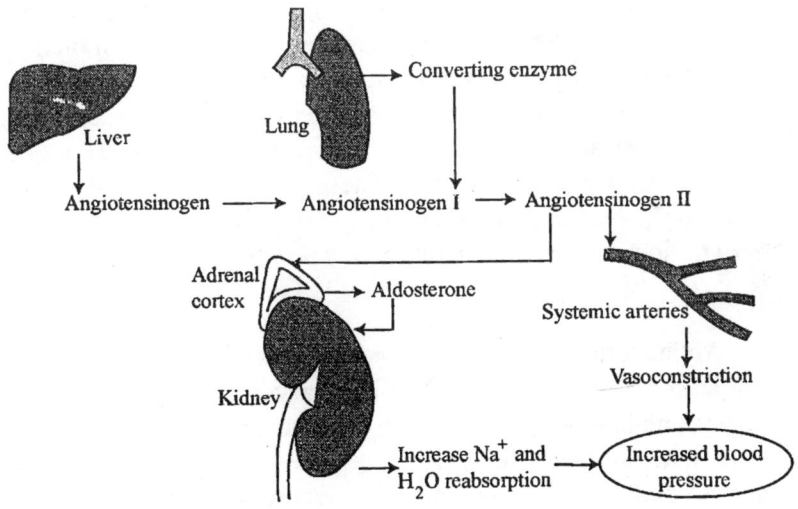

Fig. 1. Activity of angiotensinogen in relation to increased blood pressure.

Clinical Uses

Antihypertensive are used in the treatment of hypertension. Although many antihypertensive drugs are available, not all drugs may work equally well in a given patient. In some instances, the primary care provider may find it necessary to prescribe a different antihypertensive drug when the patient experiences no response to therapy. Some antihypertensive drugs are used only in severe cases of hypertension and when other less potent drugs have failed to lower the blood pressure. At times, two antihypertensive drugs may be given together to achieve a better response. Diazoxide (Hyperstat IV) and nitroprusside (Nitropress) are examples of intravenous (IV) drugs that may be used to treat hypertensive emergencies. A hypertensive emergency is a case of extremely high blood pressure that does not respond to conventional antihypertensive drug therapy.

ADVERSE REACTION

When any antihypertensive drug is given, postural or orthostatic hypotension may be seen in some patients, especially early in therapy. **Postural hypotension** is the occurrence of dizziness and light-headedness when the individual rises suddenly from a lying or sitting position. **Orthostatic hypotension** occurs when the individual has been standing in one place for a long time. These reactions can be avoided or minimized by having the patient rise slowly from a lying or sitting position and by avoiding standing in one place for a prolonged period.

Cautions

Antihypertensive drugs are used cautiously in patients with renal or hepatic impairment or electrolyte imbalances, during lactation and pregnancy, and in older patients. ACE inhibitors are used cautiously in patients with sodium depletion, hypovolemia, or coronary or cerebrovascular insufficiency and those receiving diuretic therapy or dialysis. The angiotensin II receptor agonists are used cautiously in patients with renal or hepatic dysfunction, hypovolemia, or volume or salt depletion, and patients receiving high doses of diuretics.

3.2 CONGESTIVE HEART FAILURE

The cardiotonics are drugs used to increase the efficiency and improve the contraction of the heart muscle, which leads to improved blood flow to all tissues of the body. The drugs have long been used to treat congestive heart failure (CHF), a condition in which the heart cannot pump enough blood to meet the tissue needs of the body. While the term "congestive heart failure" continues to be used by some, a more accurate term is simply "heart failure."

About 4.5 million Americans have heart failure (HF). It is the most frequent cause of hospitalization for individuals older than 65 years. Some patients, with treatment, may lead nearly normal lives, whereas more than 50% of individuals with severe HF die each year. HF is a complex clinical syndrome that can result from any number of cardiac or metabolic disorders such as ischemic heart disease, hypertension, or hyperthyroidism. Any condition that impairs the ability of the ventricle to pump blood can lead to HF. In HF, the heart fails in its ability to pump enough blood to meet the needs of the body or can do so only with an elevated filling pressure. Recently it was discovered that HF causes a number of neurohormonal changes as the body tries to compensate for the increased workload of the heart.

The sympathetic nervous system increases the secretions of the catecholamines (neurohormones epinephrine and norepinephrine), which results in increased heart rate and vasoconstriction. The activation of the Renin Angiotensin-Aldosterone (RAA) system occurs because of decreased perfusion to the kidneys. As the RAA system is activated, increased levels of angiotensin II and aldosterone occur, which increases the blood pressure, adding to the workload of the heart. These increases in neurohormonal activity cause a remodeling (restructuring) of the cardiac muscle cells, leading to hypertrophy of the heart, increased need for oxygen, and cardiac necrosis, which worsens the HF. The tissue of the heart is changed in a manner to increase the cellular mass of cardiac tissue, change the shape of the ventricle(s), and reduce the heart's ability to contract effectively.

Heart failure is best described as denoting the area of initial ventricle dysfunction: left-sided (left ventricular) dysfunction and right-sided (right ventricular) dysfunction. Left ventricular dysfunction leads to pulmonary symptoms such a dyspnea and moist cough. Right ventricular dysfunction leads to neck vein distention, peripheral edema, weight gain, and hepatic engorgement. Because both sides of the heart work together, ultimately both sides are affected in HF. Typically the left side of the heart is affected first, followed by right ventricular involvement.

The most common symptoms associated with HF include:

Left Ventricular Dysfunction

- Shortness of breath with exercise or difficulty breathing when lying flat

- Dry, hacking cough or wheezing

- Orthopnea (difficulty breathing while lying flat)

- Restlessness and anxiety

Right Ventricular Dysfunction

- Swollen ankles, legs, or abdomen, leading to pitting edema

- Anorexia

- Nausea

- Nocturia (the need to urinate frequently at night)

- Weakness

- Weight gain as the result of fluid retention

Other symptoms include:

- Palpitations, fatigue, or pain when performing normal activities

- Tachycardia or irregular heart rate

- Dizziness or confusion

Left ventricular dysfunction, also called left ventricular systolic dysfunction, is the most common form of heart failure and results in decreased cardiac output and decreased ejection fraction (the amount of blood that the ventricle ejects per beat in relationship to the amount of blood available to eject). Typically, the ejection fraction should be greater than 60%. With, left ventricular systolic dysfunction, the ejection fraction in less than 40%, and the heart is enlarged and dilated.

Until recently, the cardiotonics and a diuretic were the treatment of choice for HF. However, other drugs such as the angiotensin-converting enzyme (ACE) inhibitors and beta blockers have become the treatment of choice during the last several years.

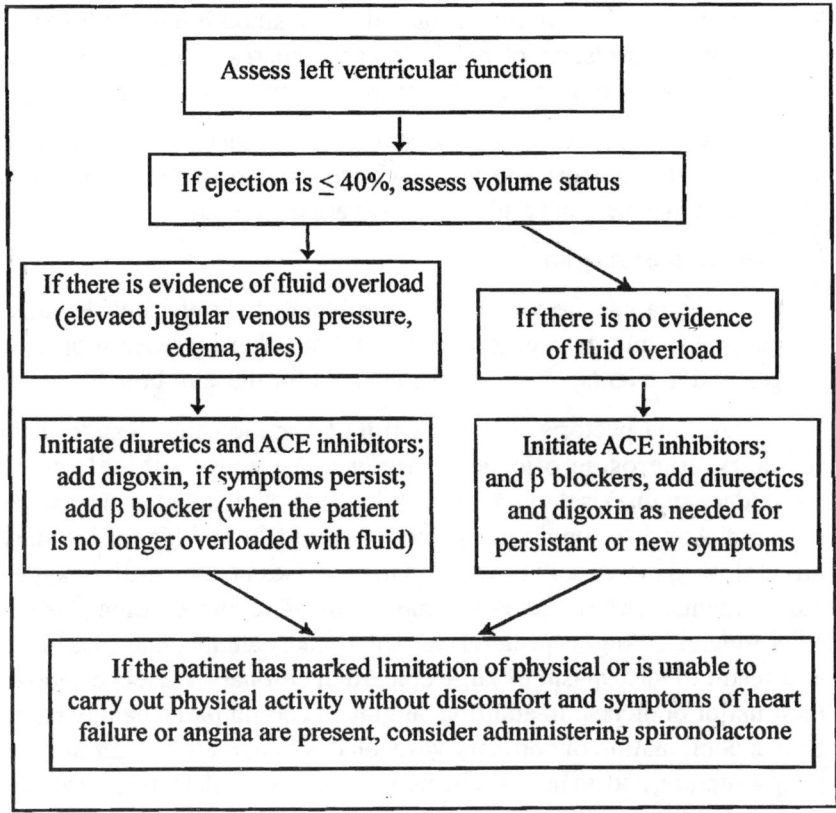

Fig. 2. Management of left ventricular systolic dysfunction.

3.3 ANGINA

Some definitions:

Atherosclerosis: Atherosclerosis is a disease characterized by deposits of fatty plaques on the inner wall of arteries. These deposits result in a narrowing of the lumen (inside diameter) of the artery and a decrease in blood supply to the area served by the artery.

Vasodilatation: Vasodilating drugs relax the smooth muscle layer of arterial blood vessels, which results in vasodilatation, an increase in the size of blood vessels, primarily small arteries and arterioles.

Angina: Angina is a disorder characterized by atherosclerotic plaque formation in the coronary arteries, which causes decreased oxygen supply to the heart muscle and results in chest pain or pressure.

Introduction of Angina:

Angina can be viewed as a problem of supply and demand. Drugs used in angina pectoris are those that either increase supply of oxygen and nutrients, or reduce the demand for these or both.

Angina pectoris is a clinical manifestation that results from coronary atherosclerotic heart disease. An acute anginal attack (secondary angina) is thought to occur because of an imbalance between myocardial oxygen supply and demand owing to the inability of coronary blood flow to increase in proportion to increases in myocardial oxygen requirements. This is generally the result of severe coronary artery atherosclerosis. Angina pectoris (variant, primary angina) may also occur as a result of vasospasm of large epicardial coronary vessels or one of their major branches. In addition, angina in certain patients may result from a combination of coronary vasoconstriction, platelet aggregation, plaque rupture, and an increase in myocardial oxygen demand (crescendo or unstable angina).

Antianginal drugs relieve chest pain or pressure by dilating coronary arteries, increasing the blood supply to the myocardium.

Supply can be increased by: cardiac work and myocardial oxygen need by:

- Dilating coronary arteries

- Slowing the heart (coronary flow, uniquely, occurs in diastole, which lengthens as heart rate falls).

Demand can be reduced by:

- Reducing afterload, (i.e. peripheral resistance), so reducing the work of the heart in perfusing the tissues.

- Reducing preload, (i.e. venous filling pressure); according to Starling's Law of the heart, workload and therefore oxygen demand varies with stretch of cardiac muscle fibres.

- Slowing the heart.

Three groups of pharmacological agents have been shown to be effective in reducing the frequency, severity, or both of primary or secondary angina. These agents include the Nitrates, β-Adrenoceptor antagonists and Calcium entry blockers.

The Therapeutic Objectives in the Use of Antianginal Drugs

The major therapeutic objectives in the treatment of angina are aimed at terminating or preventing an acute attack and increasing the patient's exercise capacity. These objectives can be achieved by reducing overall myocardial oxygen demand or by increasing oxygen supply to ischemic areas. A decrease in myocardial oxygen demand can be attained through use of the organic nitrates, calcium entry blockers, and β-adrenoceptor blocking agents. Increases in myocardial oxygen supply are more difficult to achieve, especially when coronary blood vessels are partially or totally obstructed. However, redistribution of blood flow to the subendocardium of ischemic areas has been documented in experimental animals following nifedipine (*Adalat, Procardia*), diltiazem (*Cardizem*), verapamil (*Calan*), amlodipine (*Norvasc*), nitroglycerin (*Nitrostat, Tridil, Nitro-Dur*), or propranolol (*Inderal*) administration. Increases in collateral flow to ischemic areas also have been observed in experimental animals and humans after treatment with certain calcium entry blockers and organic nitrates.

When coronary vasospasm occurs, the balance between oxygen supply and demand can be restored by relieving the spasm, thereby restoring normal coronary blood flow. Acute vasospasm has been successfully aborted through the use of nitroglycerin. In contrast, calcium entry blockers and long-acting nitrates have proved effective in the chronic therapy of coronary vasospasm.

➤ **Nitrates**

Mechanism of Actions

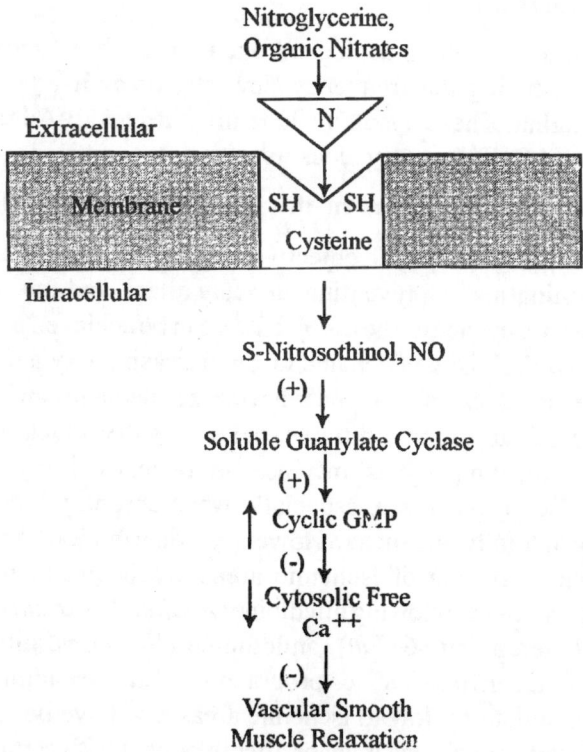

Fig. 3. Proposed mechanism by which nitroglycerin and the organic nitrates produce relaxation in vascular smooth muscle.

The nitrates, such as isosorbide (Isordil) and nitroglycerin, have a direct relaxing effect on the smooth muscle layer of blood vessels. The result of this effect is an increase in the lumen of the artery or arteriole and an increase in the amount of blood flowing through these vessels. An increased blood flow results in an increase in the oxygen supply to surrounding tissues.

Proposed mechanism by which nitroglycerin and the organic nitrates produce relaxation in vascular smooth muscle. Nitrates induce endothelial cells to release nitric oxide or a nitrosothiol (endothelium-derived releasing factor, or EDRF). EDRF activates the enzyme guanylate cyclase, which causes the generation of cyclic guanosine monophosphate (GMP), producing a decrease in cytosolic free calcium.

Clinical Uses

Sublingual or buccal nitroglycerin is used either to terminate an acute attack of angina or for short-term prevention of angina. Nitroglycerin is also the mainstay of therapy for relieving acute coronary vasospasm because of its rapid onset of action. When taken at the onset of chest pain, the effects of nitroglycerin appear within 2 to 5 minutes; however, the true duration of action is difficult to establish in patients with secondary angina, since the onset of pain causes patients to reduce their physical activity, and this alone can ameliorate the symptoms. Isosorbide dinitrate and pentaerythritol tetranitrate also can be taken sublingually, shortly before anticipated physical or emotional stress, to prevent anginal attacks.

Nitroglycerin ointment applied to the skin acts within 15 minutes and may produce its effects for 2 to 6 hours. Sustained-release transdermal nitroglycerin has been shown to deliver an antianginal effect for 2 to 4 hours following small doses and up to 24 hours after larger doses.

Orally administered long-acting nitrates, including nitroglycerin and various nitrate esters, nitroglycerin ointment, and transdermal nitroglycerin, were developed with the goal of providing a nitrate preparation that would have prolonged pharmacological activity for prophylactic therapy of angina pectoris. Considerable controversy surrounds the therapeutic use of the orally active agents because of their extensive first-pass metabolism, and many clinicians consider them to be ineffective. More recently, however, numerous clinical investigations have demonstrated the efficacy of transdermal nitroglycerin, although tolerance can be a problem with prolonged transdermal exposure to nitroglycerin. The drugs and dosage forms of organic nitrates available for therapeutic use, their usual dose, onset of action, and duration of action are summarized in Table 2.

Table 2. Dosage Forms and Pharmacokinetics of Nitrates Most Commonly Used in Angina Pectoris

Drug and Dosage Form	Usual Dose (mg)	Onset of Action (min)	Duration of Action (hr)
Nitroglycerin			
Sublingual	0.3-0.6	2-5	0.16-0.50
Transmucosal (buccal)	1-3	2-5	3-6
Oral	3-20	20-45	2-8
Ointment (2%)	1-5 (0.5-2 inches)	15-60	3-8
Transdermal	5-30 (per 24 hr)	30-60	12-24
Intravenous	5-300 mEq/min	Immediate	Transient
Isosorbide dinitrate			
Sublingual	2.5-10	3-20	1-2
Oral, chewable	5-60	30-60	2-10
Oral, sustained release	40	30-60	6-10
Isosorbide mononitrate			
Oral	20	15-30	6-12
Erythrityl tetranitrate			
Sublingual	5-10	5-15	2-3
Oral, chewable	10-30	30	2-6
Pentaerythritol tetranitrate			
Oral	10-20	30	2-6
Oral, sustained release	30-80	30-60	4-12

Adverse Effects

Vascular headache, postural hypotension, and reflex tachycardia are common side effects of organic nitrate therapy. Fortunately, tolerance to nitrate-induced headache develops after a few days of therapy. Postural hypotension and tachycardia can be minimized by proper dosage adjustment and by instructing the patient to sit down when taking rapidly acting preparations. An effective dose of nitrate usually produces a fall in upright systolic blood pressure of 10 mm Hg and a reflex rise in heart rate of 10 beats per minute. Larger changes than these should be avoided, because a reduction in myocardial perfusion and an increase in cardiac oxygen requirements may actually exacerbate the angina. Since nitrite ions oxidize the iron atoms of hemoglobin and convert it to methemoglobin, there may be a loss in oxygen delivery to tissues. While methemoglobinemia does not follow therapeutic doses of organic nitrates, it can be observed after over dosage or accidental poisoning.

Chest pain that is not relieved by two or three tablets within 30 minutes may be due to an acute myocardial infarction. In addition, nitrate administration may result in an increase in intracranial pressure, and therefore, these drugs should be used cautiously in patients with cerebral bleeding and head trauma.

> ➤ β-Adrenoceptor Blocking Agents

β-Adrenoceptor blockade is a rational approach to the treatment of angina pectoris, since an increase in sympathetic nervous system activity is a common feature in acute anginal attacks. Based on their ability to reduce oxygen demand, all β-blockers tested so far have also been shown to be effective in the treatment of secondary angina. Administration of these compounds results in a decrease in frequency of anginal attacks, a reduction in nitroglycerin consumption, an increased exercise tolerance on the treadmill, and a decreased magnitude of ST segment depression on the electrocardiogram during exercise. Propranolol is the prototype of this class of compounds.

β-Blockers approved for clinical use in secondary angina in the United States include propranolol and nadolol (*Corgard*), compounds that block both β_1- and β_2-adrenoceptors equally, while atenolol (*Tenormin*) and metoprolol (*Lopressor*) are cardioselective β_1-receptor antagonists.

Mechanism of Action

The myocardial response to exercise includes an increase in heart rate and myocardial contractility. These effects are mediated in part by the sympathetic nervous system. Propranolol and other β-adrenoceptor blockers antagonize the actions of catecholamines on the heart and thereby attenuate the myocardial response to stress or exercise. The resting heart rate is reduced by propranolol, but not to the same extent as is the decrease in exercise-induced tachycardia. Overall, propranolol reduces myocardial oxygen consumption for a given degree of physical activity.

Arterial blood pressure (afterload) is also reduced by propranolol. Although the mechanisms responsible for this antihypertensive effect are not completely understood, they are thought to involve (1) a reduction in cardiac output, (2) a decrease in plasma renin activity, (3) an action in the central nervous system, and (4) a resetting of the baroreceptors .Thus, propranolol may exert a part of its beneficial effects in secondary angina by decreasing three of the major determinants of myocardial oxygen demand, that is, heart rate, contractility, and systolic wall tension.

Propranolol and other β-blockers also have been shown to produce an increase in oxygen supply to the subendocardium of ischemic areas. The mechanism responsible for this effect is most likely related to the ability of β-blockers to reduce resting heart rate and increase diastolic perfusion time. Because subendocardial blood flow and flow distal to severe coronary artery stenosis occur primarily during diastole, this increase in diastolic perfusion time, due to the bradycardiac effect of propranolol and other β-blockers, would be expected to increase subendocardial blood flow to ischemic regions. β-Blockers have no significant effect on coronary collateral blood flow. Finally, there is evidence that β-blockers can inhibit platelet aggregation.

Clinical Uses

By attenuating the cardiac response to exercise, propranolol and other β-blockers increase the amount of exercise that can be performed before angina develops. Although propranolol does not change the point of imbalance between oxygen supply and demand at which angina occurs, it does slow the rate at which the imbalance point is reached.

Propranolol is particularly indicated in the management of patients whose angina attacks are frequent and unpredictable despite the use of organic nitrates. Propranolol may be combined with the use of nitroglycerin, the latter drug being used to control acute attacks of angina. The combined use of propranolol and organic nitrates theoretically should enhance the therapeutic effects of each and minimize their adverse effects.

Propranolol and nadolol also have been used successfully in combination with certain calcium entry blockers, particularly nifedipine, for the treatment of secondary angina. Caution should be used, however, when combining a β-blocker and a calcium channel blocker, such as verapamil or diltiazem, since the negative inotropic and chronotropic effects of this combination may lead to severe bradycardia, arteriovenous nodal block, or decompensated congestive heart failure.

Table 3. Provide additional details concerning the most commonly used β-blockers (i.e., propranolol, nadolol, atenolol, and metoprolol) in the treatment of angina pectoris.

Table 3. Doses and Pharmacokinetics of β-Receptor Antagonists Used in the Treatment of Angina Pectoris

Compound	Usual Daily Dose (mg)	Oral Bio-availability (%)	Plasma $t_{1/2}$ (hr)	First-pass Metabolism (%)
Propranolol	40-80	25-30	3-6	90
Nadolol	40	30-40	12-24	0
Metoprolol	50-100	40-45	3-4	50
Atenolol	50	50-55	5-10	0

Adverse Effects

Abrupt interruption of propranolol therapy in individuals with angina pectoris has been associated with reappearance of angina, acute myocardial infarction, or death due to a sudden increase in sympathetic nervous system tone to the heart. The mechanisms underlying these reactions are unknown, but they may be the result of an increase in the number of β-receptors that occur following chronic β-adrenoceptor blockade (up-regulation of receptors). When it is advisable to discontinue propranolol administration, such as before coronary bypass surgery, the dosage should be tapered over 2 to 3 days.

> **Calcium Channel Blockers**

Systemic and coronary arteries are influenced by movement of calcium across cell membranes of vascular smooth muscle. The contractions of cardiac and vascular smooth muscle depend on movement of extracellular calcium ions into these walls through specific ion channels. Calcium channel blockers, such as amlodipine (Norvasc), diltiazem (Cardizem), nicardipine (Cardene), nifedipine (Procardia), and verapamil (Calan), inhibit the movement of calcium ions across cell membranes. This results in less calcium available for the transmission of nerve impulses (Fig. 4). This drug action of the calcium channel blockers (also known as slow channel blockers) has several effects on the heart, including an effect on the smooth muscle of arteries and arterioles. These drugs dilate coronary arteries and arterioles, which in turn deliver more oxygen to cardiac muscle. Dilation of peripheral arteries reduces the workload of the heart. The end effect of these drugs is the same as that of the nitrates.

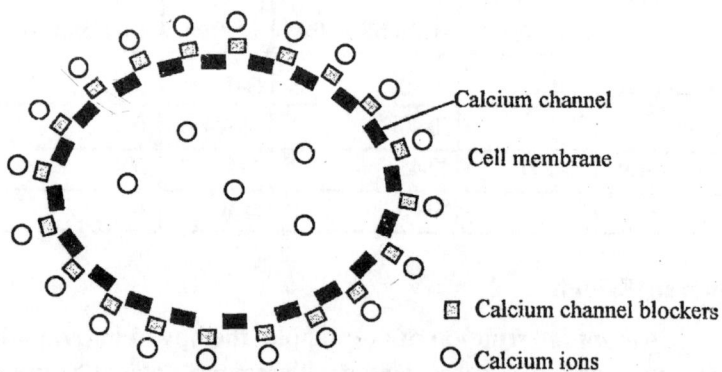

Fig. 4. Calcium channel blockers inhibit the movement of calcium ions across the cell membrane. When calcium channels are blocked by drug molecules, muscle contraction is decreased, causing the smooth muscles of the arteries and arterioles to dilate.

Clinical Uses

Calcium channel blockers are primarily used to prevent anginal pain associated with certain forms of angina, such as vasospastic (Prinzmetal's variant) angina and chronic stable angina. They are not used to abort (stop) anginal pain once it has occurred. When angina is caused by coronary artery spasm, these drugs are recommended when the patient cannot tolerate therapy with the beta β-adrenergic blocking drugs or the nitrates.

Adverse Effects

Adverse reactions to the calcium channel blocking drugs usually are not serious and rarely require discontinuation of the drug therapy. The more common adverse reactions include dizziness, light-headedness, nausea, diarrhea, constipation, peripheral edema, headache, bradycardia, flushing, dermatitis, skin rash, and nervousness.

3.4 ACUTE MYOCARDIAL INFARCTION

The incidence of coronary heart disease increases dramatically with age. Acute myocardial infarction (AMI) may present in a variety of ways in old age. Chest pain is the most common presenting symptom but atypical or silent presentations are well recognized and the incidence of painless infarction increases with advancing age. Most elderly patients with AMI have arrhythmias or conduction defects but only a minority of these are of clinical significance. The severity and mortality of AMI increase in old age. The elderly benefit as much as their younger counterparts from admission to coronary care units. Pain relief is often inadequate with opiate use and alternative drugs may be effective e.g. beta blockers, thrombolytic agents or repeated doses of nitrates. Early treatment should include streptokinase with aspirin or low dose heparin and longer term treatment in survivors should include low dose aspirin, warfarin or a beta blocker.

Classification

There are two basic types of acute myocardial infarction:

- **Transmural**: associated with atherosclerosis involving major coronary artery. It can be sub classified into anterior, posterior, or inferior. Transmural infarcts extend through the whole thickness of the heart muscle and are usually a result of complete occlusion of the area's blood supply.

- **Subendocardial**: involving a small area in the subendocardial wall of the left ventricle, ventricular septum, or papillary muscles. Subendocardial infarcts are thought to be a result of locally decreased blood supply, possibly from a narrowing of the coronary arteries. The subendocardial area is farthest from the heart's blood supply and is more susceptible to this type of pathology.

Clinically, a myocardial infarction can be further sub classified into a ST elevation MI (STEMI) versus a non-ST elevation MI (non-STEMI) based on ECG changes.

The phrase "heart attack" is sometimes used incorrectly to describe sudden cardiac death, which may or may not be the result of acute myocardial infarction. A heart attack is different from, but can be the cause of cardiac arrest, which is the stopping of the heartbeat, and cardiac arrhythmia, an abnormal heartbeat. It is also distinct from heart failure, in which the pumping action of the heart is impaired; severe myocardial infarction may lead to heart failure, but not necessarily.

A 2007 consensus document classifies myocardial infarction into five main types:

- Type 1 - Spontaneous myocardial infarction related to ischaemia due to a primary coronary event such as plaque erosion and/or rupture, fissuring, or dissection

- Type 2 - Myocardial infarction secondary to ischaemia due to either increased oxygen demand or decreased supply, e.g. coronary artery spasm, coronary embolism, anaemia, arrhythmias, hypertension, or hypotension

- Type 3 · Sudden unexpected cardiac death, including cardiac arrest, often with symptoms suggestive of myocardial ischaemia, accompanied by presumably new ST elevation, or new LBBB, or evidence of fresh thrombus in a coronary artery by angiography and/or at autopsy, but death occurring before blood samples could be obtained, or at a time before the appearance of cardiac biomarkers in the blood

- Type 4 - Associated with coronary angioplasty or stents:
  - Type 4a - Myocardial infarction associated with PCI
  - Type 4b - Myocardial infarction associated with stent thrombosis as documented by angiography or at autopsy
- Type 5 - Myocardial infarction associated with CABG.

Acute Myocardial Infarction in the Elderly

The incidence of heart disease increases with age and heart disease remains the single most important cause of death in old age, worldwide. Coronary heart disease (CHD) is the most prevalent form of cardiac disease and the incidence of this disorder increases dramatically with age.

Risk Factors for CHD

It appears that the prognostic significance of recognized risk factors for CHD is different in older people compared with the significance in younger middle aged adults. Unlike the situation in younger populations, most factors probably have a lesser effect on CHD mortality and life expectancy in affected older people compared with others of the same sex and age group'. Most of the established risk factors are, however, highly prevalent in, old age: especially high blood pressure, raised serum cholesterol, obesity, diabetes mellitus and physical inactivity.

Hypertension is a major risk factor for CHD morbidity and mortality in men and women at any age. However raised blood pressure may not be quite as important as a risk factor for cardiovascular disease over 85 years of age. The serum total cholesterol and cholesterol subfractions are predictive for CHD in older people. The adverse influence of smoking in terms of cardiovascular disease probably diminishes with age but the risk of CHD mortality increases significantly with the average daily number of cigarettes smoked and pipe-smokers or cigar smokers have CHD mortality rates which are higher than in non-smokers

Acute Myocardial Infarction

Acute myocardial infarction (AMI) may present in a variety of ways in older people. The clinical presentation may be classical. Atypical or silent (Table 4) and infarction may cause acute left ventricular failure or sudden death.

Table 4. Presentation of AMI in Old Age

Classical	Atypical	Silent
Pain Breathlessness	Acute confusion Giddiness Syncope Stroke Palpitation Abdominal Pain	No symptoms

Classical AMI is associated with crushing chest pain and/or breathlessness with sweating. Some early published studies of myocardial infarction reported a wide variation in the incidence of painless infarction in elderly people. These findings may be explained by different interpretations of what constitutes pain. The inclusion in studies of subjects unable to give a reliable history e.g. because of confusion or dysphasia and varying criteria for the actual diagnosis of myocardial infarction. Recent hospital based studies have confirmed that chest pain is present in the majority of patients over the age of 65 years with AMI. The incidence of silent AMI increases with age in both sexes. These attacks are often unrecognised but they are just as likely as recognised ones to cause strokes, heart failure or death.

Elderly, patients with AMI are more likely than younger subjects to have a history of preceding angina, hypertension, diabetes mellitus or a previous myocardial infarct. AMI should be suspected in any elderly person who has a sudden unexplained behavioral change, poor cerebral perfusion or unexplained abdominal pain or syncope.

Diagnosis

The diagnosis of myocardial infarction is made by integrating the history of the presenting illness and physical examination with electrocardiogram findings and cardiac markers (blood tests for heart muscle cell damage). A coronary angiogram allows visualization of narrowings or obstructions on the heart vessels, and therapeutic measures can follow immediately. At autopsy, a pathologist can diagnose a myocardial infarction based on anatomopathological findings.

A chest radiograph and routine blood tests may indicate complications or precipitating causes and are often performed upon arrival to an emergency. New regional wall motion abnormalities on an echocardiogram are also suggestive of a myocardial infarction. Echo may be performed in equivocal cases by the on-call cardiologist. In stable patients whose symptoms have resolved by the time of evaluation, Technetium (99mTc) sestamibi (i.e. a "MIBI scan") or thallium-201 chloride can be used in nuclear medicine to visualize areas of reduced blood flow in conjunction with physiologic or pharmacologic stress. Thallium may also be used to determine viability of tissue, distinguishing whether non-functional myocardium is actually dead or merely in a state of hibernation or of being stunned.

WHO criteria formulated in 1979 has classically been used to diagnose MI; a patient is diagnosed with myocardial infarction if two (probable) or three (definite) of the following criteria are satisfied:

1. Clinical history of ischaemic type chest pain lasting for more than 20 minutes

2. Changes in serial ECG tracings

3. Rise and fall of serum cardiac biomarkers such as creatine kinase-MB fraction and troponin

The WHO criteria were refined in 2000 to give more prominence to cardiac biomarkers. According to the new guidelines, a cardiac troponinrise accompanied by either typical symptoms, pathological Q waves, ST elevation or depression or coronary intervention are diagnostic of MI.

After Hospital Discharge

Elderly patients and their relatives are often unduly pessimistic about their recovery chances after AMI. Older post infarct patients have an increased tendency to continuing disability, especially anxiety. Breathlessness and fatigue which leads to poor exercise tolerance. Aftercare is as important as important as acute management in coronary syndromes in old people.

Patients should be firmly advised to stop smoking tobacco in any form as it is probably not safe to smoke pipes or cigars. Established hypertension in subjects up to 80 years of age should be controlled gradually to target standing blood pressures of 160/90. There is as yet no evidence of benefit to support the active lowering of raised serum cholesterol levels over 65 years of age in either sex. Physical activity should be encouraged. Suitable forms of exercise include brisk walking, swimming and cycling. Formal cardiac rehabilitation exercise programmes can be successful in selected older people after AMI. There are no recommended special diets but weight reduction should be attempted in overweight patients.

Four groups of drugs have been advocated in the secondary prevention of AMI: - anticoagulants, beta blockers, antiplatelet agents and calcium channel blockers.

The overall benefits of long-term oral anticoagulant therapy are not clear. In one study a reduced mortality rate and reinfarction rate were reported over a two year period after AMI in selected elderly patients with good anticoagulant control.

One study of long-term beta blocker therapy using alprenolol showed no benefits in older post infarct patients but a further trial of timolol did demonstrate significant reductions, compared with placebo, in overall mortality, cardiac deaths, sudden deaths and reinfarctions in men up to 75 years of age.

Aspirin will reduce vascular mortality after AMI and daily low doses should be considered in all older patients, without contraindications, who have survived an infarct. The optimum dose of aspirin has not yet been established but one recommended regimen is 162.5 mg daily.

A recent overview of all major trials of currently available calcium channel blockers has demonstrated that these agents have no special role in secondary prevention in AMI.

3.5 CARDIAC ARRHYTHMIAS

The antiarrhythmic drugs are primarily used to treat cardiac arrhythmias. A cardiac arrhythmia is a disturbance or irregularity in the heart rate, rhythm, or both, which requires administration of one of the antiarrhythmics drugs. Some examples of cardiac arrhythmias are listed in Table 5.

Table 5. Types of Arrhythmias

Arrhythmia	Description
Atrial flutter	Rapid contraction of the atria (up to 300 bpm) at a rate too rapid for the ventricles to pump efficiently
Atrial fibrillation	Irregular and rapid atrial contraction, resulting in a quivering of the atria and causing an irregular and inefficient ventricular contraction
Premature ventricular contractions	Beats originating in the ventricles instead of the sinoatrial node in the atria, causing the ventricles to contract before the atria and resulting in a decrease in the amount of blood pumped to the body
Ventricular tachycardia	A rapid heartbeat with a rate of more than 100 bpm, usually originating in the ventricles
Ventricular fibrillation	Rapid disorganized contractions of the ventricles resulting in the inability of the heart to pump any blood to the body, which will result in death unless treated immediately

An arrhythmia may occur as a result of heart disease or from a disorder that affects cardiovascular function. Conditions such as emotional stress, hypoxia, and electrolyte imbalance also may trigger an arrhythmia. An electrocardiogram (ECG) provides a record of the electrical activity of the heart. Careful interpretation of the ECG along with a thorough physical assessment is necessary to determine the cause and type of arrhythmia. The goal of antiarrhythmic drug therapy is to restore normal cardiac function and to prevent life-threatening arrhythmias.

Mechanism of Actions

The cardiac muscle (myocardium) has attributes of both nerve and muscle and therefore has the properties of both. Some cardiac arrhythmias are caused by the generation of an abnormal number of electrical impulses (stimuli). These abnormal impulses may come from the sinoatrial node or may be generated in other areas of the myocardium. The antiarrhythmic drugs are classified according to their effects on the action potential of cardiac cells and their presumed mechanism of action. As understanding of the pathophysiology of cardiac arrhythmias and the drugs used to treat these arrhythmias has increased, a method of classification has been developed that includes four basic classifications and several subclasses.

Classification of Antiarrhythmic Drugs

This is partially based on the phases of the cardiac cycle depicted in Fig. 5.

Phase 0 is the rapid depolarisation of the cell membrane that is associated with a fast inflow of sodium ions through channels that are selectively permeable to these ions.

Phase 1 is short initial period of rapid repolarisation brought about mainly by an outflow of potassium ions.

Phase 2 is a period when there is a delay in repolarisation caused mainly by a slow movement of calcium ions from the exterior into the cell through channels that are selectively permeable to these ions ('long-opening' or L-channels).

Phase 3 is a second period of rapid repolarisation during which potassium ions move out of the cell.

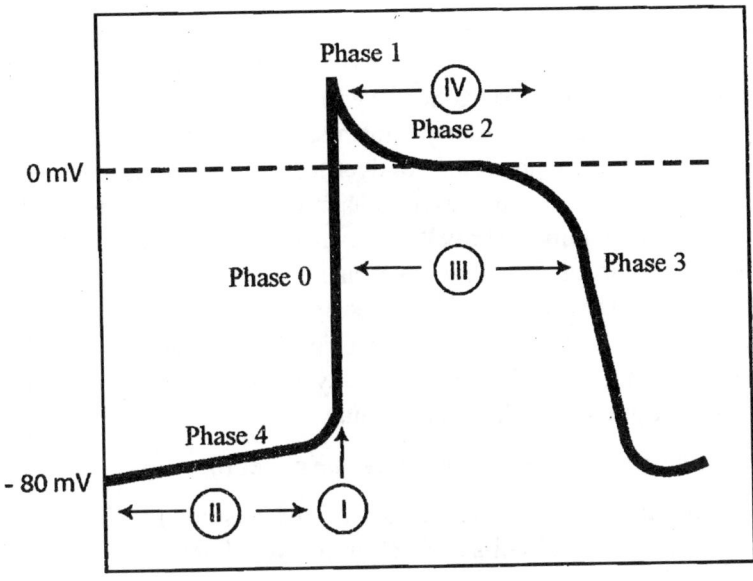

Fig. 5. The action potential of a cardiac cell that is capable of spontaneous depolarisation (SA or AV nodal, or His-Purkinje) indicating phases 0-4; the figure illustrates the gradual increase in transmembrane potential (mV) during phase 4; cells that are not capable of spontaneous depolarisation do not exhibit increase in voltage during this phase. The modes of action of antiarrhythmic drugs of classes I, II, III and IV are indicated in relation to these phases.

Phase 4 begins with the fully repolarised state; for cells that discharge *automatically*, potassium ions then progressively move back into and sodium and calcium ions move out of the cell. The result is that the interior becomes gradually less negative until a (threshold) potential is reached which allows rapid depolarisation (phase 0) to occur, and the cycle is repeated. Automaticity is also influenced by prevailing sympathetic tone. Cells that do not discharge spontaneously rely on the arrival of an action potential from another cell to initiate depolarisation.

In phases 1 and 2 the cell is in an *absolutely refractory* state and is incapable of responding further to any stimulus but during phase *3*, the relative refractory period, the cell will depolarise again if a stimulus is sufficiently strong. The orderly transmission of an electrical impulse (action potential) throughout the conducting system may be retarded in an area of disease, e.g. localised ischaemia or previous myocardial infarction. Thus an impulse travelling down a normal Purkinje fibre may spread to an adjacent fibre that has transiently failed to transmit, and pass up it in reverse direction. If this retrograde impulse should in turn re-excite the cells that provided the original impulse, a *re-entrant excitation* becomes established and may cause an arrhythmia, e.g. paroxysmal supraventricular tachycardia.

Most cardiac arrhythmias are probably due either to:

• *Impaired conduction* in part of the system leading to the formation of re-entry circuits (> 90% of tachycardias).

• *Altered rate of spontaneous discharge* in conducting tissue. Some ectopic pacemakers appear to depend on adrenergic drive.

Classification of Drugs

The Vaughan-Williams2 classification of antiarrhythmics drugs is the most commonly used classification. Despite its many peculiarities the classification does provide a useful shorthand for referring to particular groups or actions of drugs.

Class I: sodium channel blockade. These drugs restrict the rapid inflow of sodium during phase 0 and thus slow the maximum rate of depolarisation. Another term for this property is *membrane stabilising activity;* it may contribute to stopping arrhythmias by limiting the responsiveness to excitation of cardiac cells. The class may be sub classified as follows:

A. Drugs that *lengthen* action potential duration and refractoriness (adjunctive class III action), e.g. quinidine, disopyramide, procainamide.

B. Drugs that *shorten* action potential duration and refractoriness, e.g. lignocaine (lidocaine) and mexiletine.

C. Drugs that have *negligible* effect on action potential duration and refractoriness, e.g. flecainide, propafenone.

One value of the classification is that drugs in class IB are ineffective for supraventricular arrhythmias, whereas they all have some action in ventricular arrhythmias. The classification is not useful in explaining why the classes differ anatomically in their efficacy.

Class II: catecholamine blockade. Propranolol and other β-adrenoceptor antagonists reduce background sympathetic tone in the heart, reduce automatic discharge (phase 4) and protect against adrenergically stimulated ectopic pacemakers.

Class III: lengthening of refractoriness (without effect on sodium inflow in phase 0). Prolongation of the cardiac action potential and increased cellular refractoriness beyond a critical point may stop a reentrant circuit being completed and thereby prevent or halt a re-entrant arrhythmia, e.g. amiodarone and sotalol. These drugs act by inhibiting I_{Kr}, the rapidly activating component of the delayed rectifier potassium current (phase 3). The gene, *HERG* (the *human ether-à-go-go-related gene)* encodes a major subunit of the protein responsible for I_{Kr}. These are the most commonly used antiarrhythmics drugs at this time; new agents in this class include dofetilide and azimilide.

Class IV: calcium channel blockade. These drugs depress the slow inward calcium current (phase 2) and prolong conduction and refractoriness particularly in the SA and AV nodes, which may explain their effectiveness in terminating paroxysmal supraventricular tachycardia, e.g. verapamil. Although the antiarrhythmics have been entered into this classification according to a characteristic major action, most have other effects as well. For example, quinidine (class I) has major class III effects; propranolol (class II) has minor class I effects, and sotalol (class II) has major class III effects. Amiodarone has class I, II, III and IV effects but is usually classed under III.

Clinical Uses

In general these drugs are used to prevent and treat cardiac arrhythmias, such as premature ventricular contractions (PVCs), ventricular tachycardia (VT), premature atrial contractions (PACs), paroxysmal atrial tachycardia (PAT), atrial fibrillation, and atrial flutter. Some of the antiarrhythmic drugs are used for other conditions. For example, propranolol, in addition to its use as an antiarrhythmic, may also be used for patients with myocardial infarction. This drug has reduced the risk of death and repeated myocardial infarctions in those surviving the acute phase of a myocardial infarction. Additional uses include control of tachycardia in those with pheochromocytoma (a tumor of the adrenal gland that secretes excessive amounts of norepinephrine), migraine headaches, angina pectoris caused by atherosclerosis, and hypertrophic subaortic stenosis.

Adverse Effects

General adverse reactions common to most antiarrhythmics drugs include light-headedness, weakness, hypotension, bradycardia, and drowsiness. All antiarrhythmic drugs may cause new arrhythmias or worsen existing arrhythmias, even though they are administered to resolve an existing arrhythmia. This phenomenon is called the **proarrhythmic effect.** This effect ranges from an increase in frequency of premature ventricular contractions (PVCs), to the development of more severe ventricular tachycardia, to ventricular fibrillation, and may lead to death. Proarrhythmic effects may occur at any time but occur more often when excessive dosages are given, when the preexisting arrhythmia is life-threatening, or if the drug is given IV.

PART B CNS DISORDERS

3.6 EPILEPSY

Epilepsy (or epilepsies, since markedly different clinical entities exist) is a common neurological abnormality affecting about 1% of the human population. Epilepsy is a chronic, usually life-long disorder characterized by recurrent seizures or convulsions and usually, episodes of unconsciousness and/or amnesia. Followings are the major types of epileptic seizures.

Major Seizure Types

I. Partial (focal, local) seizures

    a) Simple partial seizures

    b) Complex partial seizures (psychomotor epilepsy, temporal lobe epilepsy)

    c) Partial seizures evolving to secondary generalized seizures

II. Generalized seizures

    a) Absence seizures (petit mal epilepsy)

    b) Myoclonic seizures

    c) Clonic seizures

    d) Tonic seizures

    e) Tonic-clonic seizures (grand mal epilepsy)

    f) Atonic seizures (astatic)

Patients often exhibit more than one type. In most instances, the cause of the seizure disorder is not known (idiopathic epilepsy), although trauma during birth is suspected of being one cause.

Head trauma, meningitis, childhood fevers, brain tumors, and degenerative diseases of the cerebral circulation are conditions often associated with the appearance of recurrent seizures that may require treatment with anticonvulsant drugs. Seizures also may be a toxic manifestation of the action of central nervous system (CNS) stimulants and certain other drugs. Seizures often occur in hyperthermia (febrile seizures are very common in infants); sometimes in eclampsia, uremia, hypoglycemia, or pyridoxine deficiency; and frequently as a part of the abstinence syndrome of individuals physically dependent on CNS depressants.

The therapeutic goal in epilepsy treatment is complete seizure control without excessive side effects. The prognosis depends in part upon the type of seizure disorder, but overall, only about 40 to 60% of patients become totally seizure free with available drugs. These agents are chemically and pharmacologically diverse, having in common only their ability to inhibit seizure activity without impairing consciousness. The choice of drug or drugs used depends on seizure classification, since a particular drug may be more or less specific for a particular type of seizure; patients having a mixture of seizure types present particular therapeutic difficulties. It is not always clear when to treat with one drug (monotherapy) or more than one drug (polytherapy) in a particular patient. Approximately 25% of patients given a single anticonvulsive agent do not achieve successful seizure control because of an unacceptable level of side effects. Therefore, two or more drugs may be combined in an attempt to provide better seizure control.

Convulsive disorders often begin in childhood, and drug therapy must be continued for decades; therefore, any adverse reaction is especially significant. Acknowledge of interactions between anticonvulsants and other drugs are necessary, since the patient usually must continue anticonvulsant medication regardless of the need for other drugs. Since it may be dangerous to withdraw anticonvulsant medication from a pregnant woman with epilepsy, the teratogenic potential of anticonvulsant drugs also is a consideration in the treatment of women of childbearing age.

Mechanism of Action

In epilepsy certain neurons and/or groups of neurons become hyper excitable and begin firing bursts of action potentials that propagate in a synchronous manner to other brain structures (and in the case of generalized seizures, to practically all areas of the brain). These may be the result of abnormalities in neuronal membrane stability or in the connections among neurons. It is known that the epileptic bursts consist of sodium dependent action potentials and a calcium-dependent depolarizing potential.

Recent drug development studies have centered on the capacity of known antiepileptic drugs (AEDs) to interact with ion channels, and it is now established that several agents appear to be exerting their effects primarily by inhibiting ion channels. Modulation of neuronal sodium channels decreases cellular excitability and the propagation of nerve impulses. Inhibition of sodium channels appears to be a major component of the mechanism of action of several anticonvulsant drugs.

Much interest is also centered on the role of calcium channels in neuronal activity, since the depolarization associated with burst firing is mediated by the activation of calcium channels. At therapeutically relevant concentrations, the antiabsence drug ethosuximide appears to exert its effect by inhibiting the T-type calcium channels. A portion of valproic acid's activity may also be attributable to this effect.

Table 6. Categorization of Anticonvulsants by Their Proposed Mechanism

Class	Description	Drugs
Type I	Block SRF by enhancing sodium channel inactivation	Phenytoin, Carbamazepine, Oxcarbazepine, Lamotrigine, Felbamate
Type II	Multiple actions: enhance GABAergic inhibition, reduce T-calcium currents, and possibly block SRF	Valproic acid, Benzodiazepines, Phenobarbital, Primidone
Type III	Block T-calcium currents only	Ethosuximide, Trimethadione
Type IV	Only enhances GABAergic inhibition	Vigabatrin
Noncategorized	Has no known effect on SRF, GABAergic inhibition, or T-calcium currents	Gabapentin

Disinhibition may play an important role in the generation of epileptic seizures, since a reduction of GABAergic inhibition is necessary to produce the synchronous burst discharges in groups of cells. Compounds that antagonize the activity of GABA (picrotoxinin, penicillin C, bicuculline) are CNS convulsants, while agents that facilitate GABA's inhibition have anticonvulsant activity. Several anticonvulsant drugs act to facilitate the actions of GABA.

Excitatory neurotransmitters also may be involved in the appearance of epilepsy, since the bursting activity typically seen during epileptic discharges may be due in part to the action of glutamate acting on N-methyl-Daspartate (NMDA) receptor channels to produce depolarization. It is likely that a major part of the anticonvulsant activity of felbamate involves blockade of the NMDA receptor. Table 6. Summarizes the most likely mechanism of action associated with available anticonvulsant drugs.

General Guide to Antiepilepsy Drug Therapy

The decision whether or not to initiate drug therapy after a single seizure remains controversial since approximately 25% of patients may not have another seizure. Some advocate treatment on the basis that early initiation may improve prognosis but the matter has not yet been resolved.

• Therapy should start with a *single* well-tried and safe drug. The majority of patients (70%) can be controlled on one drug (monotherapy).

• Anticonvulsant drug treatment should be 2 Greek *katamenios,* monthly appropriate to the *type* of seizure disorder. Although some drugs have a wide spectrum of action against different seizure types, some are more specific and may even aggravate certain seizure types. Carbamazepine is a drug of first choice for focal and secondary generalised epilepsy but aggravates myoclonic and absence seizures. Sodium valproate and Lamotrigine have a wide spectrum of action and are active against both primary and secondary generalised epilepsy.

• Choice of drug is also determined by the patient's *age* and *sex.* This is particularly true for women who prefer to avoid drugs associated with teratogenesis or that have adverse effects on their appearance, e.g. hirsutism from phenytoin.

- If the attempt to control a patient's epilepsy by use of a single drug is unsuccessful, it should be withdrawn and replaced by a *second line* drug, though these are effective in only about 10% of patients. There is little evidence that three drugs are better than two, and not much that two are better than one. More drugs often mean more adverse effects.

- *Abrupt withdrawal.* Effective therapy must never be stopped suddenly either by the doctor (carelessness) or by the patient (carelessness, intercurrent illness or ignorance), or status epilepticus may occur. But if rapid withdrawal is required by the occurrence of toxicity, a substantial dose of another antiepilepsy drug should be given at once.

- In cases where fits are liable to occur at a particular *time,* e.g. the menstrual period, dosage should be adjusted to achieve maximal drug effect at that time or drug treatment can be confined to this time. For example, in catamenial epilepsy, clobazam can be useful given only at period time.

Clinical Uses

In some cases, the patient does not respond well to one drug, and another drug or a combination of anticonvulsants must be tried. Dosage increases and decreases are often necessary during the initial period of treatment. Dosage adjustment also may be necessary during times of stress, severe illness, or when other drugs are being taken for treatment of conditions other than a seizure disorder. The miscellaneous anticonvulsants are adjuncts to the more widely used anticonvulsants. They are used in patients who have an inadequate response to other anticonvulsants.

Occasionally, **status epilepticus** (an emergency situation characterized by continual seizure activity with no interruptions) can occur. Diazepam (Valium) is most often the initial drug prescribed for this condition. However, because the effects of diazepam last less than 1 hour, a longer-lasting anticonvulsant, such as phenytoin or phenobarbital, also must be given to control the seizure activity.

3.7 PARKINSONISM

Parkinson's disease, also called paralysis agitans, is a degenerative disorder of the central nervous system (CNS). The disease is thought to be caused by a deficiency of dopamine and an excess of acetylcholine within the CNS. Parkinson's disease affects the part of the brain that controls muscle movement, causing such symptoms as trembling, rigidity, difficulty walking, and problems in balance. It is characterized by fine tremors and rigidity of some muscle groups and weakness of others. Parkinson's disease is progressive, that is the symptoms become worse over time. As the disease progresses, speech become slurred, the face has a masklike and emotionless expression, and the patient may have difficulty chewing and swallowing. The patient may have a shuffling and unsteady gait, and the upper part of the body is bent forward. Fine tremors begin in the fingers with a pill-rolling movement, increase with stress, and decrease with purposeful movement. Depression or dementia may occur, causing memory impairment and alterations in thinking.

Parkinson's disease has no cure, but the antiparkinsonism drugs are used to relieve the symptoms and assist in maintaining the patient's mobility and functioning capability as long as possible. For years, levodopa was the drug that provided the mainstay of treatment. Now, there are new drugs that are used either alone or in combination with levodopa. Entacapone (Comtan), pramipexole (Mirapex), and ropinirole (Requip) are newer drugs used in the treatment of Parkinson's disease. Drug-induced parkinsonism is treated with the anticholinergics benztropine (Cogentin) and trihexyphenidyl (Artane).

Parkinsonism is a term that refers to the symptoms of Parkinson's disease, as well as the Parkinson-like symptoms that may be seen with the use of certain drugs, head injuries, and encephalitis. Drugs used to treat the symptoms associated with parkinsonism are called antiparkinsonism drugs. As with some other types of drugs, it may be necessary to change from one antiparkinsonism drug to another or to increase or decrease the dosage until maximum response is obtained.

Objectives of Therapy

The dopaminergic/cholinergic balance may be restored by the following mechanisms.

1. Enhancement of dopaminergic activity by drugs which may:

   a) *Replenish* neuronal dopamine by supplying levodopa, which is its natural precursor; administration of dopamine itself is ineffective as it does not cross the blood-brain barrier

   b) Act as *dopamine agonists* (bromocriptine, pergolide, cabergoline, apomorphine);

   c) *Prolong* the action of dopamine through selective inhibition of its metabolism (selegiline).

   d) *Release* dopamine from stores and inhibit reuptake (Amantadine).

2. Reduction of cholinergic activity by antimuscarinic (anticholinergic) drugs; this approach is most effective against tremor and rigidity, and less effective in the treatment of bradykinesia (including iatrogenic, caused by dopamine receptor antagonists).

Both approaches are effective in therapy and may usefully be combined. It therefore comes as no surprise that drugs which prolong the action of acetylcholine (anticholinesterases) or drugs which deplete dopamine stores (reserpine) or block dopamine receptors (antipsychotics, e.g. chlorpromazine) will exacerbate the symptoms of parkinsonism or induce a parkinson-like state. Other parts of the brain in which dopaminergic systems are involved include the medulla (induction of vomiting), the hypothalamus (suppression of prolactin secretion) and certain paths to the cerebral cortex. Different effects of dopaminergic drugs can be explained by activation of these systems, namely emesis, suppression of lactation (mainly direct dopamine agonists) and occasionally psychotic illness. Classical antipsychotics (see p. 381) used to manage psychotic behaviour act by blockade of dopamine D_2 receptors and, as is to be expected, they are also antinauseant, may sometimes cause galactorrhoea, and can induce parkinsonism. Druginduced parkinsonism is alleviated by antimuscarinics, but not by levodopa or dopamine agonists, because the antipsychotics block dopamine receptors by which these drugs act. Since many antipsychotics also have some antimuscarinic activity, those with greatest efficacy in this respect, e.g. thioridazine, are the least likely to cause parkinsonism.

Mechanism of Action

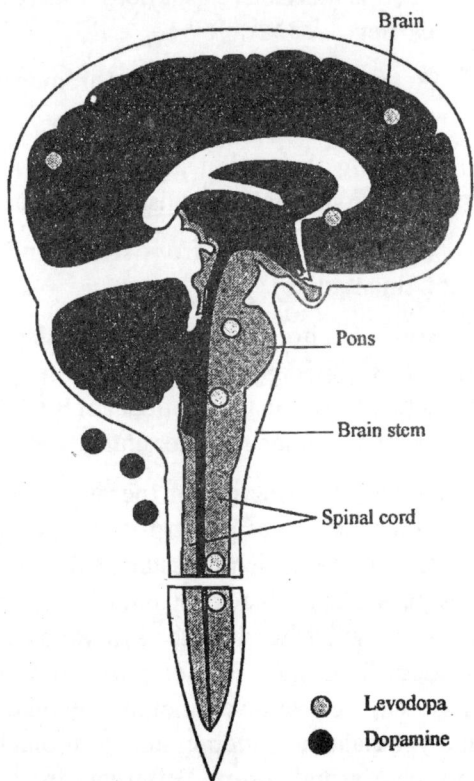

Fig. 6. The blood–brain barrier selectively inhibits certain substances from entering the interstitial spaces of the brain and spinal fluid. It is thought that certain cells within the brain form tight junctions that prevent or slow the passage of certain substances. Levodopa passes the blood–brain barrier, whereas dopamine is unable to pass.

The symptoms of parkinsonism are caused by a depletion of dopamine in the CNS. Dopamine, when given orally, does not cross the blood–brain barrier and therefore is ineffective. The body's blood–brain barrier is a meshwork of tightly packed cells in the walls of the brain's capillaries that screen out certain substances. This unique meshwork of cells in the CNS prohibits large and potentially harmful molecules from crossing into the brain. This ability to screen out certain substances has important implications for drug therapy because some drugs are able to pass through the blood–brain barrier more easily than others. Levodopa is a chemical formulation found in plants and animals that is converted into dopamine by nerve cells in the brain. Levodopa does cross the blood–brain barrier, and a small amount is then converted to dopamine. This allows the drug to have a pharmacologic effect in patients with Parkinson's disease (Fig. 6).

Combining levodopa with another drug (carbidopa) causes more levodopa to reach the brain. When more levodopa is available, the dosage of levodopa may be reduced. Carbidopa has no effect when given alone. Sinemet is a combination of carbidopa and levodopa and is available in several combinations (e.g. Sinemet 10/100 has 10 mg of carbidopa and 100 mg of levodopa; Sinemet CR is a time-released version of the combined drugs). The mechanism of action of amantadine (Symmetrel) and selegiline (Eldepryl) in the treatment of parkinsonism is not fully understood.

Uses

The dopaminergic drugs are used to treat the signs and symptoms of parkinsonism. As with some other types of drugs, it may be necessary to change from one antiparkinsonism drug to another or to increase or decrease the dosage until maximum response is obtained. Levodopa has been considered the gold standard drug therapy for Parkinson's disease since it was first used in the 1960s. Carbidopa is always given with levodopa, combined either as one drug or as two separate drugs. When it is necessary to titrate the dose of carbidopa, both carbidopa and levodopa may be given at the same time, but as separate drugs. Sometimes the response with these two drugs can be enhanced by the addition of another drug. For example, selegiline or pergolide may be added to the drug regimen of those being treated with carbidopa and levodopa but who have had a decreased response to therapy with these two drugs.

Amantadine is less effective than levodopa in the treatment of Parkinson's disease but more effective than the anticholinergics. Amantadine may be given alone or in combination with an antiparkinsonism drug with anticholinergic activity. Amantadine is also used as an antiviral drug.

Adverse Reactions

During early treatment with levodopa and carbidopa, adverse reactions are usually not a problem. But as the disease progresses, the response to the drug may become less, and the period of time that each dose is effective begins to decrease, leading to more frequent doses, and more adverse reactions.

The most serious and frequent adverse reactions seen with levodopa include **choreiform movements** (involuntary muscular twitching of the limbs or facial muscles) and dystonic movements (muscular spasms most often affecting the tongue, jaw, eyes, and neck). Less common but serious reactions include mental changes, such as depression, psychotic episodes, paranoia, and suicidal tendencies. Common and less serious adverse reactions include anorexia, nausea, vomiting, abdominal pain, dry mouth, difficulty in swallowing, increased hand tremor, headache, and dizziness. Carbidopa is used with levodopa and has no effect when given alone.

The most common serious adverse reactions to Amantadine are orthostatic hypotension, depression, congestive heart failure, psychosis, urinary retention, convulsions, leukopenia, and neutropenia. Less serious reactions include hallucinations, confusion, anxiety, anorexia, nausea, and constipation. Adverse reactions with selegiline include nausea, hallucinations, confusion, depression, loss of balance, and dizziness.

Nonpharmacological Approaches to the Treatment of Parkinsonism

Additional approaches to the treatment of Parkinson's disease include surgical procedures, brain stimulation, and transplantation of dopaminergic cells. In general, surgical procedures are reserved for patients who are refractive to levodopa or who have profound dyskinesias or fluctuations in response to levodopa. Tremor can be abolished by ablation of the ventral intermediate nucleus of the thalamus. Dyskinesias can be effectively controlled by ablation of the posteroventral portion of the globus pallidus. Brain stimulation appears to be a promising technique. High-frequency electrical stimulation of the thalamus, subthalamic nucleus, or globus pallidus can improve various symptoms of parkinsonism and reduce levodopa dosage.

A potentially promising, although very controversial, approach to the treatment of Parkinson's disease is replacement of dopaminergic neurons. The grafting of fetal substantia nigra tissue, which contains the dopamine neurons, into the striatum of parkinsonian patients has been modestly successful. The procedure will remain experimental, however, until the many practical problems and ethical issues associated with the use of fetal tissue are resolved. The discovery of pluripotent stem cells is also being viewed as a possible way of developing dopamine neurons for transplant purposes.

3.8 SCHIZOPHRENIA DEPRESSION

Schizophrenia is a group of heterogeneous, chronic psychotic disorders. Key symptoms include hallucinations, delusions, and abnormal experiences, such as the perception of loss of control of one's thoughts, perhaps to some outside entity. Patients lose empathy with others, become withdrawn, and demonstrate inappropriate or blunted mood. Discrimination of several subtypes of the disease represents only different patterns of symptoms with little value in relating behavior to neuropathology.

The disorder has a strong genetic component, as demonstrated by a concordance of 40 to 50% between monozygotic twins, but no objectiv physiological or biochemical diagnostic tests exist. Schizophrenic symptoms have been divided into two major categories. *Positive symptoms* are those that can be regarded as an abnormality or exaggeration of normal function (e.g., incoherent speech, agitation). The antipsychotic drugs are generally more effective in controlling these signs. *Negative symptoms* are those that indicate a loss or decrease in function, such as poverty of speech content or blunted affect. Both types of features are observable in most patients. Negative signs are considered to be more chronic and persistent and less responsive to some antipsychotic agents. Although any of these symptoms may undergo partial remission, persistent dysfunction and exacerbations are typical.

Schizophrenic patients appear to have small brains with large ventricular volumes, indicating a relative deficit of neurons. Structural and functional brain imaging studies have strongly suggested that regions of the medial temporal lobe (e.g., hippocampus) have diminished numbers of neurons and also have demonstrated the inability of individuals with schizophrenia to activate the frontal cortex and successfully execute tasks that require frontal cortical function. However, the relationship between behavioral signs, neuropathology, and a postulated functional excess of dopamine is unknown, and no theory of causation is conclusive.

The Dopamine Hypothesis of Schizophrenia

The dopamine hypothesis of schizophrenia is the most fully developed theory of causation for this disorder, and until recently, it has been the foundation for the rationale underlying drug therapy for this disease. The hypothesis is based on multiple lines of evidence suggesting that excessive dopaminergic activity underlies schizophrenia: (1) drugs that increase dopaminergic activity, such as levodopa and amphetamines, either aggravate existing schizophrenia or induce a psychosis indistinguishable from the acute paranoid form of the disorder; (2) traditional antipsychotic drugs strongly block D2-dopaminergic receptors in the central nervous system (CNS), and clinical efficacy is highly correlated with the potency of individual agents to bind to this receptor; (3) some postmortem studies have reported increases in dopamine receptor density in brains of schizophrenics who were not treated with antipsychotic drugs; and (4) clinical response to antipsychotic drug treatment is correlated with a decrease in homovanillic acid, a primary dopamine metabolite, in cerebrospinal fluid (CSF), plasma, and urine.

However, the dopamine hypothesis does not account for some important observations. If an abnormality of dopamine physiology were solely responsible for the pathogenesis of schizophrenia, antipsychotic drugs would do a much better job in treating patients. As it is, they are only partially effective for most and ineffective for some patients. Moreover, there is evidence that diminished glutamatergic activity also plays a role in the disease. The primary defect could emanate from nondopaminergic systems that exert a regulatory effect on dopamine neurons, leading to disinhibition of some dopaminergic pathways.

Clinical Uses

The treatment of schizophrenia is the primary indication for the use of these drugs. The principal goals for the management of a chronic schizophrenic disorder are the minimizing of symptoms and the prevention of exacerbations. Antipsychotic effectiveness is demonstrated by their ability to reduce the rate of relapse in the chronic condition by about two-thirds to three-quarters compared to no treatment. Drug choice is determined mainly by the patient's past responses and the drug's potential for producing adverse effects. The clinical trend is to prescribe the higher-potency atypical agents.

All antipsychotics except clozapine have a similar potential for producing tardive dyskinesia, the most serious adverse effect. Clozapine is reserved for patients who have failed to respond to therapy with at least two other antipsychotics and for those who have disabling tardive dyskinesia. Therapy with clozapine has been reported to salvage up to half of otherwise treatment-refractory patients. Its second-line status follows from its ability to cause seizures and a fatal agranulocytosis in large doses.

Substantial therapeutic margins exist for doses of antipsychotic drugs. Once the disorder is controlled, single daily doses are preferred. Bedtime dosing facilitates compliance and takes advantage of the sedation produced by some agents, and patients have fewer adverse reactions. Use of large doses, or rapidly increasing doses to treat severe conditions, has not proved beneficial because of the incidence of acute dystonic reactions. A parenteral form of haloperidol offers the advantage of greater bioavailability and so can be used for rapid initiation or for long-term maintenance in noncompliant individuals. During maintenance therapy, continual dosing with the smallest possible antipsychotic dose is preferred, as opposed to "as needed" treatment for recurrent episodes. Therapy is typically continued for at least a year after remissions are apparent.

Schizoaffective disorders have depression or mania as a major component in addition to psychosis. Thus, lithium or an antidepressant may have to be added to the regimen. Antipsychotic agents are also used in the initial therapy of mania because the patient's response is more rapid than with lithium. As the condition subsides, the antipsychotic can be withdrawn.

Tourette's syndrome, a heterogeneous behavioral disorder associated with motor and vocal tics of variable form and severity, can be effectively treated with haloperidol. Antipsychotics can also be employed to control disturbed behavior in senile dementia or Alzheimer's disease, since they decrease confusion, agitation, and hyperactivity. Most of these drugs also exhibit a strong antiemetic effect and can sometimes be used clinically for this purpose.

REVIEW QUESTIONS

ESSAY QUESTIONS

1.   a.Classify antihypertensive drugs.

b.Give mechanism of action and pharmacological action of methyl dopa.

2.   a.Clssify antiarrhythmic agents.

b.What are the pharmacological actions of propranolol.

c.Mechanism of action of digitalis and contra indications during digitalis therapy.

3.   Write a short note on Epilepsy.

4.   a.What is Schizophrenia?

b.Classify antipsychotic drugs.

c.Describe the pharmacological action of phenothiazines.

5.   a.Describe Parkinsonism and Classify anti- Parkinson's drugs.

b.Give the pharmacological actions of Atropine and L-Dopa.

6. a.Name the Potassium Channel blockers used as antiarrhythmic agents.

    b.Give the pharmacological action sof Quinidine and Procainamide.

7. Describe the management of Parkinsonism and the adverse reactions associated with various drugs.

SHORT ANSWER QUESTIONS

8. Describe the pharmacotherapy of Epilepsy.

9. Write about the drug therapy for Angina Pectoris.

10. What are the various drugs used in treatment of Congestive Heart failure.

11. Explain about Myocardial Infarction.

12. Describe the treatment options for bipolar depression.

13. Write short note o Proton Pump Inhibitors.

14. What are different types of psychological disorders?

15. Explain monoamine pathway theory of depression.

16. Add a note on anti depressant drugs.

Chapter 4

RESPIRATORY DISEASES

4.1 ASTHMA

Asthma is a chronic inflammatory disorder of the airways in which many cells and cellular elements play a role, in particular, mast cells, eosinophils, T lymphocytes, macrophages, neutrophils, and epithelial cells. In susceptible individuals, this inflammation causes recurrent episodes of wheezing, breathlessness, chest tightness, and coughing, particularly at night or in the early morning. These episodes are usually associated with widespread but variable airflow obstruction that is often reversible either spontaneously or with treatment. The inflammation also causes an associated increase in the existing bronchial hyper responsiveness to a variety of stimuli.

With asthma there is increasing airway obstruction caused by bronchospasm and bronchoconstriction, inflammation and edema of the lining of the bronchioles, and the production of thick mucus that can plug the airway (see Fig. 1).

There are three types of asthma:

i. Extrinsic (also referred to as allergic asthma and caused in response to an allergen such as pollen, dust, and animal dander)

ii. Intrinsic asthma (also called nonallergic asthma and caused by chronic or recurrent respiratory infections, emotional upset, and exercise)

iii. Mixed asthma (caused by both intrinsic and extrinsic factors)

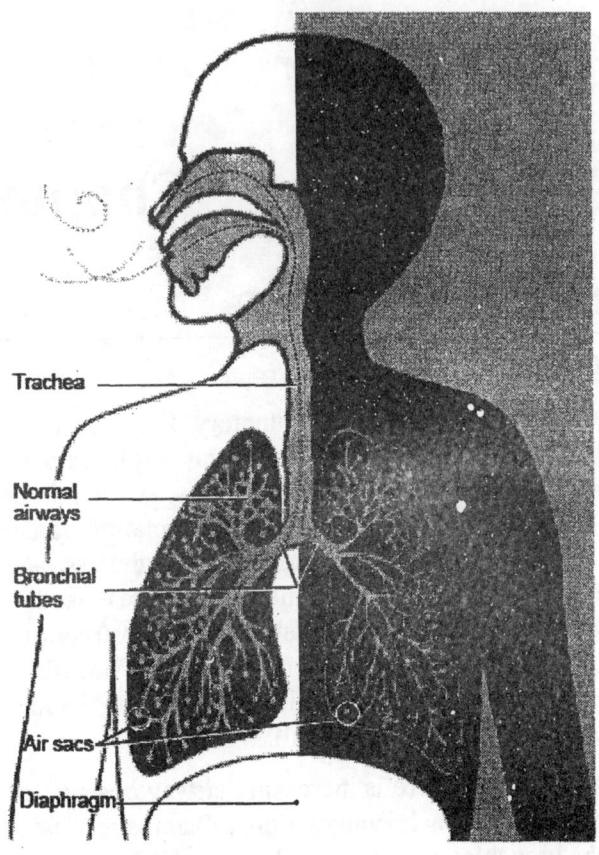

Trachea

Normal airways

Bronchial tubes

Air sacs

Diaphragm

Fig. 1. _Left column_. Normal lungs: Air comes into the body through the nose and mouth. Air then goes through the trachea pipe into all the airways. The air reaches the tiny air sacs deep in the lungs, where gas exchanges takes place.

Right column. Lungs in asthma: In asthma, the patient has trouble moving air through the lungs because airways become narrow as the muscles in their walls tighten and the airway walls swell up. The swollen walls give off extra mucus, which clogs the narrowed airways.

Extrinsic or allergic asthma causes the IgE inflammatory response. With exposure, the IgE antibodies are produced and attach to mast cells in the lung. Reexposure to the antigen causes them to bind to the IgE antibody, releasing histamine and other mast cell products. The release of these products causes bronchospasm, mucous membrane swelling, and excessive mucous production. Gas exchange is impaired, causing carbon dioxide to be trapped in the alveoli so that oxygen is unable to enter. Fig. 2 identifies the asthmatic pathway from both intrinsic and extrinsic stimulus.

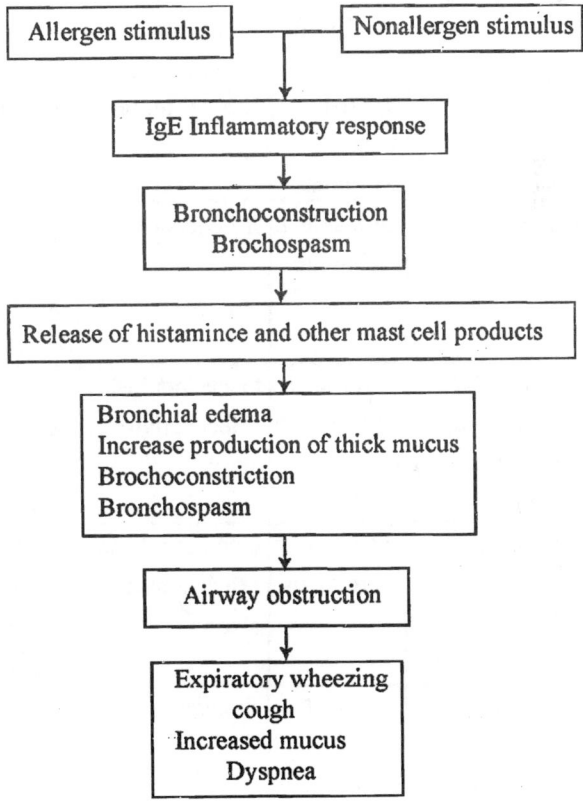

Fig. 2. Asthmatic pathway from intrinsic and extrinsic stimulus.

Other disorders of the lower respiratory tract include emphysema (lung disorder in which the terminal bronchioles or alveoli become enlarged and plugged with mucus) and chronic bronchitis (chronic inflammation and possibly infection of the bronchi). Chronic obstructive pulmonary disease (COPD) is the name given collectively to emphysema and chronic bronchitis because the obstruction to the airflow is present most of the time. Asthma that is persistent and present for most of the time may also be referred to as COPD

Classification of Asthma

Table 1. Classification of asthma in a patient with untreated, newly diagnosed asthma

	Daytime asthma symptoms	Night-time asthma symptoms	Exacerbations	Spirometry
Intermittent	Less than weekly	Less than 2 per month	Infrequent,Brief	FEV1 at least 80% predictedFEV1 variability less than 20%
Mild persistent	More than weekly and less than daily	More than 2 per month but not weekly	Occasional,May affect activity or sleep	FEV1 at least 80% predictedFEV1 variability 20–30%
Moderate persistent	Daily	Weekly or more often	Occasional,May affect activity or sleep	FEV1 60–80% predictedFEV1 variability more than 30%
Severe persistent	Daily,Physical activity is restricted	Frequent	Frequent	FEV1 60% predicted or lessFEV1 variability more than 30%

Intermittent asthma

Untreated asthma is classified as intermittent if **all** the following apply:

- Daytime asthma symptoms occur less than once per week.
- Night-time asthma symptoms occur less than twice per month.
- Exacerbations are infrequent and brief.
- FEV1 is at least 80% predicted and varies by less than 20%.

Mild persistent asthma

Untreated asthma is classified as mild persistent if **one or more** of the following applies (and more severe signs and symptoms are **not** present):

- Daytime asthma symptoms occur more than once per week but not every day.
- Night-time asthma symptoms occur more than twice per month, but not every week.
- Exacerbations occur occasionally and may affect activity or sleep.
- FEV1 is at least 80% predicted and varies by 20–30%.

Moderate persistent asthma

Untreated asthma is classified as moderate persistent if **one or more** of the following applies (and more severe signs and symptoms are **not** present):

- Daytime asthma symptoms occur every day, but do not generally restrict physical activity.
- Night-time asthma symptoms occur at least once per week.
- Exacerbations occur occasionally and may affect activity or sleep.
- FEV1 is 60–80% predicted and varies by more than 30%.

Severe persistent asthma

Untreated asthma is classified as severe persistent if **one or more** of the following applies:

- Daytime asthma symptoms occur every day and restrict physical activity.

- Night-time asthma symptoms occur every day.

- Exacerbations are frequent.

- FEV1 is 60% predicted or less, and varies by more than 30%.

Treatment Strategy

Clinical symptoms alone cannot be used as an accurate assessment of the severity of physiological impairment in the asthmatic patient, because a substantial degree of impairment may persist even after symptoms are relieved by treatment. Consequently, the overall objectives of antiasthma therapy are to return lung function to as near normal as possible and to prevent acute exacerbations of the disease. For quality of life, the ideal regimen permits normal activities, including exercise, with minimal or no side effects.

The primary classes of drugs used to treat asthma are bronchodilators and anti-inflammatory agents. Bronchodilators include theophylline, a variety of adrenomimetic amines, and ipratropium bromide. Anti-inflammatory therapy consists of the corticosteroids. A growing collection of drugs called alternative therapies cannot be classified clearly as either bronchodilators or anti-inflammatory agents. These agents include the leukotriene modulators, cromolyn sodium, and nedocromil sodium.

Bronchodilators are used both in maintenance therapy and as needed to reverse acute attacks. These agents are often referred to as **relievers** because they provide rapid symptomatic relief but do not affect the fundamental disease process. Based on the underlying pathophysiology of the disease, **anti-inflammatory** therapy must be used in conjunction with bronchodilators in all but the mildest asthmatics. Anti-inflammatory agents are also called **controllers** because they provide long-term stabilization of symptoms. In addition to drug therapy, all treatment regimens should include patient education focused on three key behaviors: (1) the appropriate use of medications to control symptoms (e.g., proper technique for use of metered-dose inhalers), (2) recognition of the signs of a deteriorating disease status (e.g., a progressive increase in the use of bronchodilators), and (3) prevention strategies (e.g., avoidance of antigenic material; influenza vaccination to forestall virus induced exacerbations).

BRONCHODILATORS

A **bronchodilator** is a drug used to relieve bronchospasm associated with respiratory disorders, such as bronchial asthma, chronic bronchitis, and emphysema. These conditions are progressive disorders characterized by a decrease in the inspiratory and expiratory capacity of the lung. Collectively, they are often referred to as COPD. The patient with COPD experiences dyspnea (difficulty breathing) with physical exertion, has difficulty inhaling and exhaling, and may exhibit a chronic cough.

The two major types of bronchodilators are the sympathomimetics and the xanthine derivatives. The anticholinergic drug ipratropium bromide (Atrovent) is used for bronchospasm associated with COPD, chronic bronchitis, and emphysema.

Bronchodilators: Sympathomimetics

Examples of sympathomimetic bronchodilators include albuterol (Ventolin), epinephrine (Adrenalin), salmeterol (Serevent), and terbutaline (Brethine). Many of the sympathomimetics used as bronchodilators have the sub classification of beta-2 (β_2) receptor agonists (e.g., albuterol, salmeterol, and terbutaline).

Actions

When bronchospasm occurs, there is a decrease in the lumen (or inside diameter) of the bronchi, which decreases the amount of air taken into the lungs with each breath. A decrease in the amount of air taken into the lungs results in respiratory distress. Use of a bronchodilating drug opens the bronchi and allows more air to enter the lungs, which in turn, completely or partially relieves respiratory distress.

USES

Sympathomimetics (drugs that mimic the sympathetic nervous system) are used primarily to treat reversible airway obstruction caused by bronchospasm associated with acute and chronic bronchial asthma, exercise-induced bronchospasm, bronchitis, emphysema, bronchiectasis (abnormal condition of the bronchial tree), or other obstructive pulmonary diseases.

Adverse Reactions

Administration of a sympathomimetic bronchodilator may result in restlessness, anxiety, increase in blood pressure, palpitations, cardiac arrhythmias, and insomnia. When these drugs are used by inhalation, excessive use (e.g., over the recommended times) may result in paradoxical bronchospasm.

Bronchodilators: Xanthine Derivatives

Examples of the **xanthine derivatives** (drugs that stimulate the central nervous system [CNS] resulting in bronchodilation, also called methylxanthines) are theophylline and aminophylline.

Actions

The xanthine derivatives, although a different class of drugs, also have bronchodilating activity by means of their direct relaxation of the smooth muscles of the bronchi.

Uses

The xanthine derivatives are used for symptomatic relief or prevention of bronchial asthma and reversible bronchospasm associated with chronic bronchitis and emphysema.

Adverse Reactions

Adverse reactions associated with administration of the xanthine derivatives include nausea, vomiting, restlessness, nervousness, tachycardia, tremors, headache, palpitations, increased respirations, fever, hyperglycemia, and electrocardiographic changes.

ANTIASTHMA DRUGS

Asthma is a respiratory condition characterized by recurrent attacks of dyspnea (difficulty breathing) and wheezing caused by spasmodic constriction of the bronchi. With asthma, the body responds with a massive inflammation. During the inflammatory process, large amounts of histamine are released from the mast cells of the respiratory tract, causing symptoms such as increased mucous production and edema of the airway and resulting in bronchospasm and inflammation. With asthma the airways become narrow, the muscles around the airway tighten, the inner lining of the bronchi swell, and extra mucus clogs the smaller airways. (See Fig. 1.)

Along with the bronchodilators, several types of drugs are effective in the treatment of asthma. These include corticosteroids, leukotriene formation inhibitors, leukotriene receptor agonists, and mast cell stabilizers.

Antiasthma drugs are used in various combinations to treat and manage asthma. Using several drugs may be more beneficial than using a single drug. A multidrug regimen allows smaller dosages of each drug, decreasing the number and severity of adverse reactions.

Antiasthma Drugs: Corticosteroids

Actions

Corticosteroids, such as beclomethasone (Beclovent), flunisolide (AeroBid), and triamcinolone (Azmacort), are given by inhalation and act to decrease the inflammatory process in the airways of the patient with asthma. In addition, the corticosteroids increase the sensitivity of the β_2-receptors. With increased sensitivity of the β_2-receptors, the β_2-receptor agonist drugs are more effective.

Uses

The corticosteroids are used in the management and prophylactic treatment of the inflammation associated with chronic asthma or allergic rhinitis.

Adverse Reactions

When used to manage chronic asthma, the corticosteroids are most often given by inhalation. Adverse reactions to the corticosteroids are less likely to occur when the drugs are given by inhalation rather than taken orally. Occasionally, patients may experience throat irritation causing hoarseness, cough, or fungal infection of the mouth and throat. Vertigo or headache also may occur.

Antiasthma Drugs: Leukotriene Receptor Antagonists and Leukotriene Formation Inhibitors

Leukotriene receptor antagonists include montelukast sodium (Singulair) and zafirlukast (Accolate). Zileuton (Zyflo) is classified as a leukotriene formation inhibitor.

Actions

Leukotrienes are bronchoconstrictive substances released by the body during the inflammatory process. When leukotriene production is inhibited, bronchodilation is facilitated. Zileuton acts by decreasing the formation of leukotrienes. Although the result is the same, montelukast and zafirlukast work in a manner slightly differently from that of zileuton. Montelukast and zafirlukast are considered leukotriene receptor antagonists because they inhibit leukotriene receptor sites in the respiratory tract, preventing airway edema and facilitating bronchodilation.

Uses

Zafirlukast and zileuton are used in the prophylaxis and treatment of chronic asthma in adults and children older than 12 years. Montelukast is used in the prophylaxis and treatment of chronic asthma in adults and in children older than 2 years.

Adverse Reactions

Adverse reactions of zafirlukast (Accolate) include headache, dizziness, myalgia, pain, nausea, diarrhea, abdominal pain, vomiting, and fever. Montelukast (Singulair) administration may cause headache, dizziness, dyspepsia, flu-like symptoms, cough, abdominal pain, and fatigue. Adverse reactions seen with the administration of zileuton (Zyflo) include dyspepsia, nausea, abdominal pain, and headache. Liver enzyme elevations may occur with the administration of zileuton. These elevations may continue to rise, remain unchanged, or resolve with continued therapy. Alanine aminotransferase (ALT) is an enzyme produced by the liver that acts as a catalyst in the transamination reaction necessary for amino acid production. ALT is found in liver cells in high concentration. When liver damage occurs, ALT levels increase, which makes ALT testing a valuable test for monitoring liver function.

Antiasthma Drugs: Mast Cell Stabilizers

Mast cell stabilizers include cromolyn sodium (Intal) and nedocromil sodium (Tilade).

Actions

These drugs inhibit the release of substances that cause bronchoconstriction and inflammation from the mast cells in the respiratory tract.

Uses

The mast cell stabilizers are used in combination with other drugs in the treatment of asthma and other allergic disorders, including allergic rhinitis (nasal solution), and in the prevention of exercise-induced bronchospasm. When the mast cell stabilizers are used in conjunction with other antiasthma drugs, a reduction in dosage of the drugs may be possible after using the mast cell stabilizer for 3 or 4 weeks. These drugs may be given by nebulization, aerosol spray, or as an oral concentrate.

Adverse Reactions

The more common adverse reactions associated with the mast cell stabilizers include headache, dizziness, nausea, fatigue, hypotension, or unpleasant taste in the mouth. These drugs may cause nasal or throat irritation when given intranasally or by inhalation.

GASTROINTESTINAL DISORDERS

4.2 PEPTIC ULCER DISEASE

Peptic ulcer disease is defined as pathological lesions and ulcer of any portion of the gastro-intestinal tract exposed to acid activated pepsin and result from imbalanced between the erosive action of acid and pepsin on one hand and the gastro-duodenal mucosal defense system on the other. Although high acid output appears to be an important causative factor. In duodenal ulcer, it cannot explain the environment of ulcer in every patient. Nocturnal acid secretion, rather than total acid output, appears to be of particular importance in the pathogenesis of duodenal bicarbonate secretion. In patients with gastric ulcers, on the other hand, acid output is normal or reduced, which suggest that altered mucosal resistance is a primary factor in development of ulcer.

There are three groups of factor which are related to production of ulceration.

1. Genetic Factors: Hydrochloric acid, Pepsin, Reflux Bile, NSAIDS, Alcohol, Pancreatic Proteolytic enzymes, Bacterial Toxin.

2. Defensive Factors: Mucus, Bicarbonates, Blood flow, Restitution of epithelium.

3. Role of *Helicobacter pylori* (*H.pylori*): Helicobacter pylori appear to be a major cause of chronic type B antral gastritis. The evidence for such a link in peptic ulcer is less clear. Although *H.pylori* has been identified in more than 955 of patients with duodenal ulcer and in 60% to 70% of those with gastric ulcer, its role in the development of acid peptic disorder is ulcertain because it is also present in a significant percentage of asymptomatic disorder.

The causes & mechanisms of formation of Peptic ulcer

The peptic ulcer is an excoriated area of the mucosa caused by the digestive action of gastric juice. The most common site of peptic ulcer is the pyloric region of duodenum. In addition peptic ulcers frequently occur along the lesser curvature of the stomach or more rarely in the lower end of the oesophasgus, where stomach juice frequently refluxes.

Basic causes of peptic ulceration

The usual cause of peptic ulceration is much secretion of gastric juice in relation to the degree of protection afforded to the mucus by the mucus that is also secreted by the mucus cells.

Use of Aspirin, Non-steroidal anti-inflammatory drugs (NSAIDS), smoking, genetic factors and environmental influences also may contribute to the development of chronic peptic ulcer.

Mechanism of peptic ulceration:

The mechanisms by which the peptic ulcer is formed are described as below:

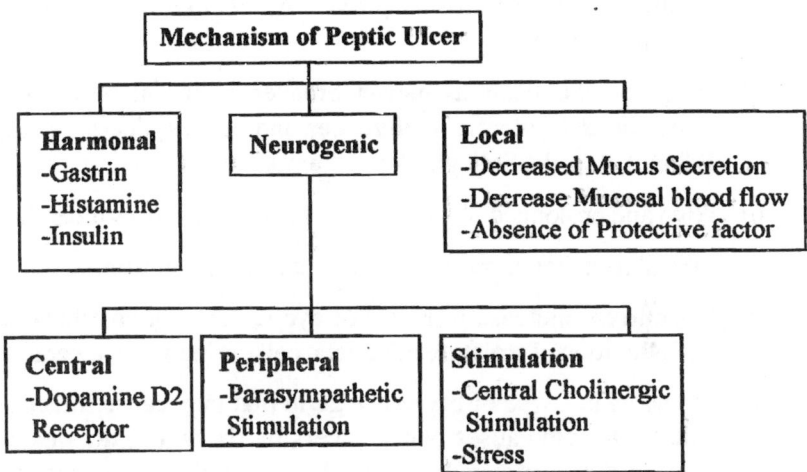

Mechanisms:

a) Excess stimulation of dorsal motor nucleus of the vagus by impulses originating in the cerebrum causes ulceration.

b)   The reduction of endogenous prostaglandin biosynthesis in the lumen of duodenum. Prostaglandins are agents protecting the integrity of duodenal mucosa against injury from luminal contents. Thus Indomethacin, Indoxol, Phenylbutazone induce ulcer by inhibiting the prostaglandin synthesis.

c)   Disruption of gastric mucosal barrier to back diffusion of H^+ is a postulation and considered as an etiologic factor for stress induced ulceration.

d)   The decrease in rectal temperature increases the incidence of gastric ulceration.

e)   Undampered oscillation of central cholinergic system causes ulceration E.g. by shock.

f)   Less bold supply to a local area of stomach or duodenal causes ulceration because this area becomes unable to secret the required protective juices. This is proved by occlusion of superior mesenteric artery.

g)   Drugs or chemicals as barrier breaker by initial decrease in transmucosal potential differences and causes ulceration E.g. Ethanol, Aspirin, Salicylic Acid, thermal injury.

h)   High and prolonged blood levels of Histamine causes ulceration.

i)   Stimulation of central D2-receptor causes ulceration.

j)   Concurrent increase in levels of cyclic-AMP in gastric tissue and alteration of structure of parietal cell during stress ulceration.

k)   *H. pylori* is   pe of bacteria a germ that may cause infection. The bacterium causes peptic ulcers by damaging the mucous coating that protects the stomach and duodenum. Damage to the mucous coating allows powerful stomach acid to get through to the sensitive lining beneath. Together, the stomach acid and *H. pylori* irritate the lining of the stomach or duodenum and cause an ulcer[1].

Symptoms:

> ➤ Abdominal discomfort is the most common symptom. Thi⸱ discomfort usually

- Is a dull, gnawing ache.
- Comes and goes for several days or weeks.
- Occurs 2 to 3 hours after a meal.
- Occurs in the middle of the night (when the stomach is empty).
- Is relieved by food.
- Is relieved by antacid medications.

> ➤ **Other symptoms include**

- weight loss
- poor appetite
- bloating
- burping
- nausea
- vomiting

Some people experience only very mild symptoms or none at all.

> ➤ **Emergency Symptoms**

- Sharp, sudden, persistent stomach pain
- Bloody or black stools
- Bloody vomit or vomit that looks like coffee grounds

They could be signs of a serious problem, such as

- **Perforation:** Sometimes an ulcer eats a hole in the wall of the stomach or duodenum, and bacteria and partially digested food can spill through the opening into the sterile abdominal cavity (peritoneum) and cause peritonitis, an inflammation of the abdominal cavity and wall.

- **Bleeding:** As an ulcer eats into the muscles of the stomach or duodenal wall, blood vessels may also be damaged, causing bleeding.

- **Obstruction:** Ulcers located at the end of the stomach, where the duodenum is attached, can cause swelling and scarring, which can narrow or close the intestinal opening. This obstruction can prevent food from leaving the stomach and entering the small intestine, resulting in vomiting the contents of the stomach.

Diagnosis Tests for Peptic Ulcer:

The list of tests used in the diagnosis of Peptic Ulcer includes:

- **Blood test:** This test checks for the presence of H. pylori antibodies. A disadvantage of this test is that it sometimes can't differentiate between past exposure and current infection. Additionally, a false-negative is possible if you've recently been taking certain drugs, such as antibiotics or proton pump inhibitors.

- **Breath test:** This procedure uses a radioactive carbon atom to detect H. pylori. For the test, you drink a small glass of clear, tasteless liquid. The liquid contains radioactive carbon as part of a substance (urea) that will be broken down by H. pylori. Less than an hour later, you blow into a bag, which is then sealed. If you're infected with H. pylori, your breath sample will contain the radioactive carbon in the form of carbon dioxide. The advantage of the breath test is that it can monitor the effectiveness of treatment used to eradicate H. pylori, detecting whether the bacteria have been killed or eradicated.

- **Stool antigen test:** This test checks for H. pylori in stool samples. It's useful both in helping to diagnose H. pylori infection and in monitoring the success of treatment.

- **Upper gastrointestinal (upper GI) X-ray:** This test outlines your esophagus, stomach and duodenum. During the X-ray, you swallow a white, metallic liquid (containing barium) that coats your digestive tract and makes an ulcer more visible. An upper GI X-ray can detect some ulcers, but not all.

- **Endoscopy:** This procedure may follow an upper GI X-ray if the X-ray suggests a possible ulcer, or doctor may perform endoscopy first. In this more sensitive procedure, a long, narrow tube with an attached camera is threaded down your throat and esophagus into your stomach and duodenum. With this instrument, your doctor can view your upper digestive tract and identify an ulcer. Your doctor will perform this test if you have other signs or symptoms, such as difficulty swallowing, weight loss, vomiting (particularly vomiting red or black material that looks like coffee grounds), black stools or anemia.

Complications

If ulcers remain untreated they may lead to:

- Bleeding

- Perforation (an actual puncture through the stomach)

- Obstruction (repeated attacks may cause scar tissue that can block the digestive tract)

Treatment of Peptic Ulcer

- Medications: medications that decrease the amount of acid produced by the stomach are used to provide quick pain relief and promote rapid healing.

- Other equally effective medications, such as coating agents called carafate, antacids, and one called omeprazole, are available.

- Most peptic ulcers heal within 4 to 6 weeks of treatment. Take your medications regularly as directed, otherwise your ulcer may not heal completely and your symptoms could return. Symptoms may disappear in a few days, but DO NOT STOP taking your medication.

- Nighttime is the most important time to heal ulcers, since many people produce large amounts of stomach acid while they sleep. Take antacids as needed between meals and at bedtime to neutralize stomach acid and reduce pain.

- Aspirin and anti-inflammatory products should be avoided. Let your doctor know if you have been taking these, so alternate medications may be prescribed.

- Side effects from the medication used to treat peptic ulcer disease are very infrequent (less than 5 percent), but many include mild diarrhea, dizziness, nausea, drowsiness, rash or headache.

- Remember, people are different and no single medicine is best for everyone. If your symptoms worsen, notify your doctor immediately.

4.3 ULCERATIVE COLITIS

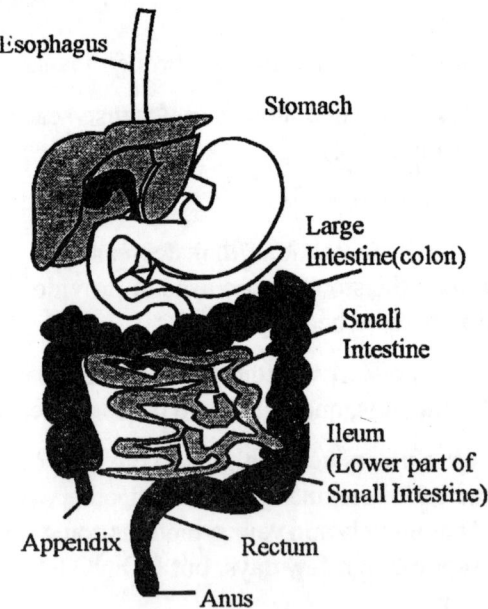

The Gastrointestinal Tract

Fig.3. Ulcerative colitis

Ulcerative colitis is a disease that causes inflammation and sores, called ulcers, in the lining of the rectum and colon. Ulcers form where inflammation has killed the cells that usually line the colon, then bleed and produce pus. Inflammation in the colon also causes the colon to empty frequently, causing diarrhea.

The inflammation in ulcerative colitis usually begins in the rectum and lower colon, but it also may involve the entire colon. Ulcerative colitis may be called by other names, depending on where the disease is located in the colon.

- **Ulcerative proctitis:** involves only the rectum.

- **Proctosigmoiditis:** affects the rectum and sigmoid colon (the lower segment of the colon before the rectum).

- **Distal colitis:** involves only the left side of the colon.

- **Pancolitis:** affects the entire colon.

Ulcerative colitis is an inflammatory bowel disease (IBD), the general name for diseases that cause inflammation in the small intestine and colon. It can be difficult to diagnose because its symptoms are similar to other intestinal disorders and to another type of IBD called Crohn's disease. Crohn's disease differs because it causes inflammation deeper within the intestinal wall and can occur in other parts of the digestive system including the small intestine, mouth, esophagus, and stomach.

Ulcerative colitis can occur in people of any age, but it usually starts between the ages of 15 and 30, and less frequently between 50 and 70 years of age. It affects men and women equally and appears to run in families, with reports of up to 20 percent of people with ulcerative colitis having a family member or relative with ulcerative colitis or Crohn's disease. A higher incidence of ulcerative colitis is seen in Whites and people of Jewish descent.

What are the symptoms of ulcerative colitis?

The most common symptoms of ulcerative colitis are abdominal pain and bloody diarrhea. Patients also may experience

- Anemia
- Fatigue
- Weight loss
- Loss of appetite
- Rectal bleeding
- Loss of body fluids and nutrients
- Skin lesions
- Joint pain
- Growth failure (specifically in children)

About half of the people diagnosed with ulcerative colitis have mild symptoms. Others suffer frequent fevers, bloody diarrhea, nausea, and severe abdominal cramps. Ulcerative colitis may also cause problems such as arthritis, inflammation of the eye, liver disease, and osteoporosis. It is not known why these problems occur outside the colon. Scientists think these complications may be the result of inflammation triggered by the immune system. Some of these problems go away when the colitis is treated.

Causes of Ulcerative Colitis

Many theories exist about what causes ulcerative colitis. People with ulcerative colitis have abnormalities of the immune system, but doctors do not know whether these abnormalities are a cause or a result of the disease. The body's immune system is believed to react abnormally to the bacteria in the digestive tract.

Ulcerative colitis is not caused by emotional distress or sensitivity to certain foods or food products, but these factors may trigger symptoms in some people. The stress of living with ulcerative colitis may also contribute to a worsening of symptoms.

Diagnosis

Many tests are used to diagnose ulcerative colitis. A physical exam and medical history are usually the first step.

Blood tests may be done to check for anemia, which could indicate bleeding in the colon or rectum, or they may uncover a high white blood cell count, which is a sign of inflammation somewhere in the body.

A stool sample can also reveal white blood cells, whose presence indicates ulcerative colitis or inflammatory disease. In addition, a stool sample allows the doctor to detect bleeding or infection in the colon or rectum caused by bacteria, a virus, or parasites.

A colonoscopy or sigmoidoscopy are the most accura.e methods for making a diagnosis of ulcerative colitis and ruling-out other possible conditions, such as Crohn's disease, diverticular disease, or cancer. For both tests, the doctor inserts an endoscope (a long, flexible, lighted tube connected to a computer and TV monitor) into the anus to see the inside of the colon and rectum. The doctor will be able to see any inflammation, bleeding, or ulcers on the colon wall. During the exam, the doctor may do a biopsy, which involves taking a sample of tissue from the lining of the colon to view with a microscope.

Sometimes x rays such as a barium enema or CT scans are also used to diagnose ulcerative colitis or its complications.

Treatment for Ulcerative Colitis

Treatment for ulcerative colitis depends on the severity of the disease. Each person experiences ulcerative colitis differently, so treatment is adjusted for each individual.

Drug Therapy

The goal of drug therapy is to induce and maintain remission, and to improve the quality of life for people with ulcerative colitis. Several types of drugs are available.

- Aminosalicylates, drugs that contain 5-aminosalicyclic acid (5-ASA), help control inflammation. Sulfasalazine is a combination of sulfapyridine and 5-ASA. The sulfapyridine component carries the anti-inflammatory 5-ASA to the intestine. However, sulfapyridine may lead to side effects such as nausea, vomiting, heartburn, diarrhea, and headache. Other 5-ASA agents, such as olsalazine, mesalamine, and balsalazide, have a different carrier, fewer side effects, and may be used by people who cannot take sulfasalazine. 5-ASAs are given orally, through an enema, or in a suppository, depending on the location of the inflammation in the colon. Most people with mild or moderate ulcerative colitis are treated with this group of drugs first. This class of drugs is also used in cases of relapse.

- Corticosteroids such as prednisone, methylprednisone, and hydrocortisone also reduce inflammation. They may be used by people who have moderate to severe ulcerative colitis or who do not respond to 5-ASA drugs. Corticosteroids, also known as steroids, can be given orally, intravenously, through an enema, or in a suppository, depending on the location of the inflammation. These drugs can cause side effects such as weight gain, acne, facial hair, hypertension, diabetes, mood swings, bone mass loss, and an increased risk of infection. For this reason, they are not recommended for long-term use, although they are considered very effective when prescribed for short-term use.

- Immunomodulators such as azathioprine and 6-mercapto-purine (6- MP) reduce inflammation by affecting the immune system. These drugs are used for patients who have not responded to 5-ASAs or corticosteroids or who are dependent on corticosteroids. Immunomodulators are administered orally, however, they are slow acting and it may take up to 6 months before the full benefit. Patients taking these drugs are monitored for complications including pancreatitis, hepatitis, a reduced white blood cell count, and an increased risk of infection. Cyclosporine A may be used with 6-MP or azathioprine to treat active, severe ulcerative colitis in people who do not respond to intravenous corticosteroids.

Other drugs may be given to relax the patient or to relieve pain, diarrhea, or infection. Some people have remissions (periods when the symptoms go away) that last for months or even years. However, most patients' symptoms eventually return.

Hospitalization

Occasionally, symptoms are severe enough that a person must be hospitalized. For example, a person may have severe bleeding or severe diarrhea that causes dehydration. In such cases the doctor will try to stop diarrhea and loss of blood, fluids, and mineral salts. The patient may need a special diet, feeding through a vein, medications, or sometimes surgery.

Surgery

About 25 to 40 percent of ulcerative colitis patients must eventually have their colons removed because of massive bleeding, severe illness, rupture of the colon, or risk of cancer. Sometimes the doctor will recommend removing the colon if medical treatment fails or if the side effects of corticosteroids or other drugs threaten the patient's health.

Surgery to remove the colon and rectum, known as proctocolectomy, is followed by one of the following:

- Ileostomy, in which the surgeon creates a small opening in the abdomen, called a stoma, and attaches the end of the small intestine, called the ileum, to it. Waste will travel through the small intestine and exit the body through the stoma. The stoma is about the size of a quarter and is usually located in the lower right part of the abdomen near the beltline. A pouch is worn over the opening to collect waste, and the patient empties the pouch as needed.

- Ileoanal anastomosis, or pull-through operation, which allows the patient to have normal bowel movements because it preserves part of the anus. In this operation, the surgeon removes the colon and the inside of the rectum, leaving the outer muscles of the rectum. The surgeon then attaches the ileum to the inside of the rectum and the anus, creating a pouch. Waste is stored in the pouch and passes through the anus in the usual manner. Bowel movements may be more frequent and watery than before the procedure. Inflammation of the pouch (pouchitis) is a possible complication.

Not every operation is appropriate for every person. Which surgery to have depends on the severity of the disease and the patient's needs, expectations, and lifestyle. People faced with this decision should get as much information as possible by talking to their doctors, to nurses who work with colon surgery patients (enterostomal therapists), and to other colon surgery patients. Patient advocacy organizations can direct people to support groups and other information resources.

4.4 HEPATITIS

The term "hepatitis" means inflammation of the liver. Hepatitis may be caused by viruses, bacteria, drugs, toxins, or excess alcohol intake. Viral hepatitis was first recognized as a distinct clinical entity during the late 18th and early 19th centuries. At that time, reports of scattered outbreaks of this syndrome, referred to as infectious hepatitis, epidemic hepatitis, or catarrhal jaundice, began to appear in the medical literature. The viruses associated with the main clinical feature of hepatitis or jaundice are known as the hepatitis viruses, of which there are currently five described - hepatitis A, B, C, E and D viruses, although other viruses can cause hepatitis as part of a wider illness, for example, CMV and EBV. There are likely to be others, as yet uncharacterized, hepatitis viruses.

Viral hepatitis is the most common of the serious contagious diseases, with significant morbidity and mortality resulting from acute illness (hepatitis A, B, C, D, E) and cirrhosis and liver cancer associated with chronic infection (hepatitis B, C, D) in addition to adverse economic effects.

Viral hepatitis can be transmitted enterically and parenterally.

Enterically Transmitted Hepatitis

This occurs when a sufficient amount of the virus enters the mouth to cause infection. This can occur through direct contact with an infected person's faeces or indirect faecal contamination of food, water supply, shellfish or utensils. This is the main route of transmission for hepatitis A and E.

Parenterally Transmitted Hepatitis

This is when the disease is transmitted from one person to another by infectious blood and body fluids. The people most likely to become infected include:

- The family of infected persons (including newborn infants)

- Injecting drug users (current or previous)

- Recipients of transfusions, blood or blood products, or transplanted organs prior to 1990 when blood banks began testing for hepatitis C

- Persons with needle-stick injury

- Institutionalized persons

- Persons with multiple sex partners

- Persons with tattoos

- Healthcare professionals - rare in the UK

Hepatitis B, C & D are transmitted parenterally, hence including them in the blood-borne viruses.

Hepatitis can be caused by:

- Toxins

- Certain drugs

- Some diseases

- Heavy alcohol use

- Bacterial and viral infections

Hepatitis is most often caused by one of several viruses, which is why it is often called viral hepatitis. The most common types of viral hepatitis in the United States are hepatitis A, hepatitis B, and hepatitis C.

Signs of Viral Hepa-titis

Some people with viral hepatitis have no signs of the infection. Symptoms, if they do appear, can include:

- Body aches, weakness, tiredness

- Loss of appetite

- Nausea or vomiting

- Diarrhea or constipation

- Dark urine

- Light colored stool

- Fever

- Headache

- A dull ache in the right upper side of the abdomen

- Jaundice, which is when the skin and whites of the eyes turn yellow

- Itchy skin

- Joint pain and rashes

Modes of Viral Hepatitis

You can get hepatitis A by eating food or drinking water contaminated with feces (stool) from a person infected with the virus or by anal-oral contact. Some ways you can get this type of hepatitis include:

- Eating food prepared by a person with the virus who didn't wash his or her hands after using the bath-room and then touched the food.

- Contact with infected household members or sexual partners.

- Touching diaper changing tables that aren't cleaned properly.

- Eating raw shellfish that came from sewage-contaminated water.

You can get hepatitis B if you come into contact with an infected person's:

- Blood

- Semen and other fluids from having sex

- Needles from drug use

The virus can also be passed from an infected mother to her baby during childbirth.

Hepatitis C is also spread through contact with the blood of an infected person. This usually happens when people use contaminated needles to inject drugs.

Diagnosis Viral Hepatitis

If you think you might have viral hepa-titis, see your doctor. To diagnose your illness, your doctor will:

- Ask you questions about your health history

- Do a physical exam

- Order blood tests

Hepatitis infections are diagnosed with blood tests that look for parts of the virus or antibodies your body makes in response to the virus.

Treatment of Hepatitis A

The treatment of acute hepatitis A is basically a common-sense regimen of adequate rest, a low fat, high carbohydrate diet, adequate fluid intake and no alcohol. Foods like fruits vegetables, breads, cereals, grains such as rice and pasta, and lean meat, chicken, fish or eggs usually cause no problems. However fatty foods such as chips, crisps, biscuits, pastries, chocolate, cream, butter, margarine and fried foods are usually not well tolerated. You are unlikely to need to be in hospital unless you are unable to keep down enough fluids and there is a danger of dehydration. There are other signs of serious liver disease such as mental confusion or abnormal blood clotting tests. The good news about hepatitis A is that a complete recovery should occur within one to two months, although occasionally recovery may take up to six months. Hepatitis A does not cause chronic infection or serious long-term liver damage, although in rare cases, it may cause severe acute hepatitis and liver failure, and even death.

Treatment of Hepatitis B

Acute hepatitis B does not need any treatment. The approach is similar to that of acute hepatitis A and involves a sensible diet without too much fat, plenty of rest and no alcohol. If symptoms are mild, you can be treated at home. If you have severe symptoms, especially jaundice, you may be treated in hospital as there is a small chance of liver failure. In some rare instances (<1%), it can lead to fulminant hepatitis and liver failure and may need a liver transplant.

Treatment for chronic hepatitis B has improved in recent times.

Treatment does not lead to a cure in most patients but it will slow the progression of disease (to prevent progression to liver cirrhosis) in most patients. Treatments available in Australia for chronic hepatitis B include lamivudine (Zeffix), adefovir (Hepsera), entecavir (Baraclude) and pegylated interferon (PEG IFN). There are also many trials involving newer antiviral agents (clevudine, tenofovir and telbivudine) that are available in some tertiary hospital liver clinics.

Patients with chronic hepatitis B are at risk of developing hepatoma (primary liver cancer) and they will need to be monitored closely with blood test (AFP—alphafoetoprotein) and ultrasound.

Vaccination is available to prevent contracting hepatitis B.

Hepatitis B vaccination was introduced to the Australian Childhood Immunisation Schedule in 2000. Adults who are at risk of contracting hepatitis B and who should be vaccinated include health care workers, intravenous drug users, prisoners, people with chronic liver disease, people working in sex industry and individuals with many sexual partners.

Treatment of Hepatitis C

The treatment of chronic hepatitis C has improved significantly in recent time. Combination therapy of pegylated interferon (Peg IFN, subcutaneous injection) and ribavirin (tablets) can lead to a cure (negative HCV RNA) in approximately 55% of patients. Patients with genotype 2 or 3 hepatitis C virus are more likely to respond (75% to 88%). Response rate for genotype I (commonest genotype in Australia) is approximately 50%.

There are many trials involving newer interferon (albuferon given fortnightly rather than weekly) or oral antiviral therapy in tertiary hospital liver clinics.

So far, there is no effective vaccine or immune globulin to prevent infection with hepatitis C.

Testing for Hepatitis A

Antibodies are proteins produced by the body's immune system to defend it against infection. In acute hepatitis A, the body produces specific antibodies (called 1gM antibodies) to defend itself against hepatitis A virus. Tests for hepatitis A infection look for these 1gM antibodies. If found, they confirm a diagnosis of acute hepatitis A.

As the acute hepatitis gets better, another type of antibody against hepatitis A virus called IgG appears and stays in the blood. If this antibody is found in your blood, it shows you once had hepatitis A infection and are now immune to further infection.

Testing for Hepatitis B

The hepatitis B virus is spherical with an outer coat and an inner core. A protein which is part of the surface coat is found in the blood of people infected with hepatitis B. This protein is called hepatitis B surface antigen or HepBsAg ('antigen' means protein component of the virus).

The body produces a number of different antibodies to hepatitis B infection which can be detected by blood tests. One of them - hepatitis B core antibody (HBcAb) - is present in the early stages of infection with the virus. It can also be detected in chronic carriers if they have a flare-up in the activity of their hepatitis. Another antibody - hepatitis B surface antibody (HBsAb) - can be detected in those who have fully recovered from hepatitis B infection. These people will be immune to further infection.

If they are immune because they have been vaccinated against hepatitis B, however, rather than acquiring the immunity from having successfully over- come infection, only hepatitis B surface antibody will be found. In neither case of immunity is hepatitis B surface antigen present in the blood.

People who are chronically infected (hepatitis B carriers) will have hepatitis B surface antigen and hepatitis B core antibodies in their blood, but no hepatitis B surface antibody. The goal of treating hepatitis B is to stop growth of the virus. Tests can now measure if the hepatitis B virus is growing actively and whether the person's blood is infectious. When the virus is actively growing, hepatitis B 'e' antigen (HBeAg) and hepatitis B DNA (HBVDNA), the genetic material of the virus, are present in blood.

When the virus stops growing, either because the immune system has overcome it, or as a result of treatment, hepatitis B 'e' antigen disappears and hepatitis B e antibody appears. Hepatitis B DNA either decreases or disappears completely.

If the virus is still present in the liver but not growing, hepatitis B surface antigen will he found in the blood but hepatitis B DNA and hepatitis B c antigen will not. There may or may not be liver damage in those with active viral growth.

	Carrier (Low infectivity)	Carrier (High infectivity)	Previous infection	Previous vaccination
HBsAG	✓	✓		
HBcAb	✓	✓	✓	
HBeAg		✓		
ABeAb	✓		✓	
HBV-DNA		✓		
HBsAb			✓	✓

So checking for the presence of these various antibodies and antigens in the blood allows doctors to see whether someone is infected with hepatitis B, whether that infection is acute or chronic, whether the person is infectious or a carrier and whether he or she is immune from further infection and why.

Testing for Hepatitis C

Tests to identify the Hepatitis C virus are not as sophisticated as for hepatitis B. Most people infected with the hepatitis C virus have hepatitis C antibody in their blood. If a blood test detects these antibodies (a positive antibody test) it indicates an earlier exposure to the virus. (Occasionally, however, low levels of antibodies will be found with no other evidence of previous infection. This is called a false positive antibody test.)

There are two different methods to detect these antibodies. One is the enzyme-linked immuno-sorbent assay (ELISA); the other is called the recombinant immuno-blot assay (MBA). The ELISA is more often used as the MBA is more expensive.

There is another test which measures the hepatitis C virus in blood or liver tissue using a technique called the polymerase chain reaction (PCR). This detects tiny amounts of the genetic material of the hepatitis C virus but it is technically difficult and is used mainly in special research laboratories.

Liver Function Tests

These help diagnose problems and estimate their severity. They also give a picture of the likely outcome, and show whether treatment is improving liver function. There is no one test that shows exactly how well the liver is working, so a number of different tests are necessary. They include the following:

Bilirubin

High levels of bilirubin usually indicate that the liver cells are functioning poorly or the bile duct is obstructed. Bilirubin comes from the breakdown of the haem pigment (the red colour) in ageing red blood cells. Red blood cells normally survive for about four months. When they reach the end of their life span, they are broken down, mainly in the spleen, and some of the by-products such as proteins and iron are recycled. The haem pigment is converted to bilirubin. The liver extracts bilirubin from the blood and passes it via the bile into the intestine from where it is excreted in faeces. There is normally some bilirubin in the blood, but if the liver is not functioning normally, bilirubin levels rise. A high blood level of bilirubin may also indicate that blood cells are being destroyed at a greater rate than normal (a process known as haemolysis), or that the flow of bile out of the liver is blocked. This can occur with cancer in the pancreas or bile duct, or if the main bile duct is blocked by gall stones, or if the small bile ducts within the liver are injured.

Serum Enzyme Tests

Tests of the level of certain enzymes in the blood usually show the type of liver injury, and whether it is due to hepatitis or to blockage to the flow of bile. However, these enzyme tests cannot distinguish one type of hepatitis from another; there are other special tests for this. The serum enzyme tests that are commonly done measure the following four enzymes:

- Aspartate aminotransferase (AST): an enzyme present in large quantities in the heart, liver, muscle and kidney. Blood levels rise when any of these tissues are acutely damaged.

- Alanine aminotransferase (ALT): an enzyme present in a greater proportion in the liver than in the heart or in muscle. A high level of this enzyme therefore measures liver cell damage more specifically than a high level of AST. A rise in the level of transaminase enzymes helps to diagnose liver cell injury due to viral hepatitis. However, other liver problems also produce high levels of these enzymes, such as damage due to sensitivity to certain drugs or if the blood supply to the liver is interrupted. So high levels of transaminase enzymes show that liver cells are damaged, but not the type of damage. Obstruction to the bile ducts usually causes only a moderate rise in levels of transaminase enzymes.

- Gamma glutamyl transpeptidase (Gamma GT): High blood levels of this enzyme may be due to hepatitis or bile duct obstruction. Levels may also be high if you've been drinking too much alcohol for too long, or are taking certain medications such as anti-convulsant drugs. Sometimes, however, gamma GT levels may be high without necessarily indicating liver problems.

- Alkaline phosphatase (ALP): The level of this enzyme rises if the bile duct is obstructed or injured by infection or medication and, to a lesser extent, when liver cells are damaged by hepatitis. High levels suggest obstruction in the bile duct, or, possibly, liver cancer. Alkaline phosphatase can also be high in some types of hepatitis when there is no blockage of the bile duct. This is known as a cholestatic form of hepatitis.

Blood Proteins

A number of important proteins are made by the liver. These include albumin, fibrinogen, and many of the blood clotting factors. Abnormal levels of these proteins are found with severe hepatitis or in chronic liver disease. The tests most useful in suggesting the cause of jaundice are the levels of serum alkaline phosphatase and serum transaminase enzymes. Repeated measurements of bilirubin, albumin, transaminases, and clotting proteins can help to assess how severe liver damage is. High levels of transaminase enzymes do not always indicate severe liver injury. Falling levels of albumin and clotting factors indicate deteriorating liver function. Liver cancer or certain infections are suggested by an isolated high serum alkaline phosphatase when other liver tests are normal.

In addition to these traditional liver function tests, there are more specific tests such as those for viral hepatitis markers and immunological tests for specific antibodies.

4.5 CIRRHOSIS

Introduction

Cirrhosis is a condition that affects the liver. The liver weighs about 3 pounds and is the largest organ in the body. It is located in the upper right side of the abdomen, below the ribs. When specific diseases cause the liver to become permanently injured and scarred, the condition is called cirrhosis.

The scar tissue that forms in cirrhosis harms the structure of the liver, blocking the flow of blood through the organ. The loss of normal liver tissue slows the processing of nutrients, hormones, drugs, and toxins by the liver. Also slowed is production of proteins and other substances made by the liver.

Cirrhosis is a leading cause of illness and death in the United States. In the United States, approximately 5.5 million people (2% of the U.S. population) are affected by cirrhosis. Cirrhosis causes 26,000 deaths each year and is the seventh leading cause of death in the United States among adults between the ages of 25 and 64. It is expected that the number of people affected by cirrhosis will continue to increase in the near future.

Cirrhosis of the liver is a consequence of long-term liver injury of many types. While excess alcohol use and chronic infection with hepatitis viruses (such as hepatitis B and hepatitis C) are the most common causes of cirrhosis in the United States, cirrhosis can be caused by other conditions including fatty liver disease, inherited disorders, drug-induced injury, bile duct disorders and autoimmune diseases. Some patients may have more than one cause for cirrhosis (such as alcohol excess and viral hepatitis). A large portion of patients (up to 20%) do not have an identifiable cause for cirrhosis. This is known as *cryptogenic cirrhosis.*

Function of the Liver

Blood from the digestive system (stomach, intestines) passes through the liver on its way back to the heart. The liver is the largest internal organ and is involved in many complex metabolic functions essential to life.

- The liver extracts nutrients from the blood and processes them for later use.

- The liver makes bile, which is used by the digestive system to help absorb fat and certain vitamins.

- The liver also removes medications and toxic waste-products from the blood and excretes them into bile.

- The liver is the body's main factory for blood proteins, including the proteins involved in normal blood clotting function. Your doctor may check blood clotting tests (prothrombin time or INR) as a measure of your liver function.

How Does Cirrhosis Develop?

There are many causes of liver injury such as excessive alcohol consumption, viruses, inherited disorders, drug-related injury and environmental toxin exposure. Injury to the liver leads to inflammation which may be detected by abnormalities in liver-related blood tests. Over time, ongoing injury leads to the development of scar tissue in the liver, a process called *fibrosis*. Since the liver has a substantial amount of reserve function, mild to moderate amounts of fibrosis usually do not lead to symptoms. However, as the amount of fibrosis increases it can lead to disruptions in the normal shape and function of the liver.

Cirrhosis occurs when the normal structure of the liver is disrupted by bands of scar tissue. One of the normal functions of the liver is to filter blood returning to the heart from the digestive system. When cirrhosis is present, the presence of scar tissue causes increased resistance to blood flow through the liver. These results in high pressures developing in the veins that drain into the liver, a process called *portal hypertension*. Many of the complications of liver disease, such as fluid retention and esophageal bleeding, are caused by the presence of portal hypertension.

Symptoms of Cirrhosis

The signs and symptoms of liver cirrhosis may be absent or non-specific at early stages. Early non-specific symptoms include fatigue and itching. As scar tissue replaces healthy tissue and liver function worsens, a variety of liver-related symptoms may develop.

- **Fatigue:** Fatigue is a common symptom of cirrhosis. Many patients with cirrhosis also develop loss of muscle mass which can worsen fatigue. Fatigue due to cirrhosis can be difficult to treat and it is important to seek out other causes of fatigue may be unrelated to liver disease.

- **Itching:** Itching (also called *pruritus*) is a common symptom of cirrhosis. Itching is most common in patients with cirrhosis due to bile duct disorders, but itching can occur in any type of liver disease. Patients with itching due to liver disease typically have itching over large parts of their body and the itching can be severe. A variety of medications can be used to treat cirrhosis-related itching.

- **Edema** is the retention of abnormal amounts of fluid in the body, most frequently in the legs.

- When significant fluid retention occurs in the abdomen (belly) this is called *Ascites.* Ascites can cause abdominal discomfort and shortness of breath when the amount of fluid is large enough to restrict the normal expansion of the chest during breathing.

- **Digestive Tract Bleeding:** Patients with cirrhosis can develop abnormally enlarged veins (*varices*) inside the digestive system. Varices typically do not cause symptoms unless they rupture and bleed. Bleeding varices can be identified by the vomiting of blood or coffee-ground-like material or the passage of maroon or black, tarry stools. Bleeding from esophageal varices is a medical emergency and requires emergency treatment in your nearest hospital.

- **Jaundice** is a yellow discoloration of the skin and whites of the eyes. Darkening of the urine (iced-tea or cola colored) and/or pale (putty-colored) stools often occurs before the yellow discoloration of the skin and whites of the eyes develops.

- Patients with cirrhosis can develop symptoms of mental slowing, confusion, excess drowsiness, and slurring of speech, a condition known as *hepatic encephalopathy.*

Diagnosis of Cirrhosis

Cirrhosis is best determined by examining a sample of liver tissue under the microscope, a procedure which is called a *liver biopsy.* In this relatively simple procedure a thin needle is inserted, under local anesthesia, into the liver and removes a small piece of liver tissue. Liver biopsy not only confirms the presence of cirrhosis, but can often provide information as to its cause.

In many cases, a liver biopsy may not be necessary to identify cirrhosis. Frequently, your physician may be able to diagnose cirrhosis by the presence of changes noted during physical examination (such as enlargement of the spleen, enlargement of the breast tissue in men, and certain skin findings) together with the results from blood tests, imaging studies (such as ultrasound, CT or MRI scans) and/or endoscopy. There are several new tests that use ultrasound or MRI to directly measure the stiffness of the liver which may help in diagnosing cirrhosis but these tests are not all widely available.

In a liver biopsy, a needle is used to take a small piece of liver tissue. That sample is then examined under a microscope.

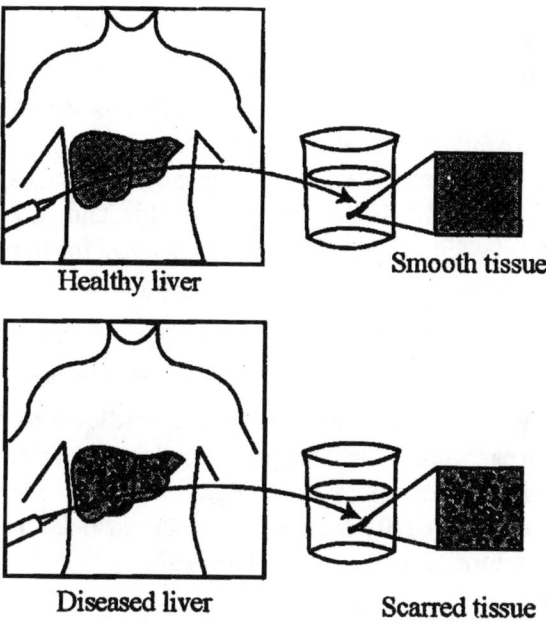

Fig .4. Cirrhosis, liver biopsy

Treatments for Cirrhosis

Medical care for patients with cirrhosis has several aims: treating the underlying cause of liver disease, preventing cirrhosis-related complications, and treating the symptoms of cirrhosis. Since cirrhosis is a chronic disease, patients with cirrhosis require ongoing medical care with a physician specializing in the care of patients with liver disease (a gastroenterologist or hepatologist).

Whenever possible, the underlying cause of cirrhosis should be treated. Some conditions improve with medial therapy and treatment can improve or delay worsening of liver function. In some circumstances, patients may not tolerate treatments for their underlying liver disease because their cirrhosis is too advanced. Patients with cirrhosis should not drink alcohol. In patients who consume alcohol regularly, liver function may improve significantly with total avoidance of alcohol.

Your doctor may recommend various treatments aimed at preventing complications of cirrhosis from developing. Infection is an important cause of illness in patients with cirrhosis and your doctor may recommend updating your vaccinations. Typically, patients with cirrhosis should receive a yearly flu (influenza) vaccine and the pneumonia (pneumococcal) vaccine. Your doctor may test you for hepatitis A and hepatitis B and vaccinate you if you are not immune.

Your doctor may prescribe various treatments to help control symptoms from complications of cirrhosis. These may include:

- Dietary salt restriction and diuretic medications (commonly known as "water pills") are prescribed for the control of ascites and edema. In some cases, a small needle may be inserted into the abdominal cavity under local anesthesia to drain ascites fluid, a procedure known as a *paracentesis.*

- Patients who have experienced prior episodes of spontaneous bacterial peritonitis are given long-term antibiotic medication to prevent future episodes.

- Various medications may be prescribed for patients with hepatic encephalopathy. These include lactulose and/or oral antibiotics. In rare cases, dietary protein restriction may be recommended.

- Patients with esophageal varices may be treated with blood-pressure reducing medications or treatment may be applied directly to the varices during an endoscopy.

In some cases your doctor may recommend the insertion of a **TIPS shunt**. The placement of a TIPS shunt is an invasive procedure. A TIPS shunt is a metal tube (also called a stent) placed within the liver under x-ray guidance through an incision in the jugular vein in the neck. TIPS shunt works by decreasing the pressure against which blood must flow within the liver (that is to reduce *portal hypertension*). TIPS shunts are used to treat patients with severe difficulty with ascites or bleeding from varices that is not able to be controlled with medication or endoscopy. Not all patients should receive a TIPS shunt. TIPS shunt insertion has associated risks and the placement of TIPS shunt can lead to new or *worsening hepatic encephalopathy*.

For some patients with severe liver disease, *liver transplantation* may be considered as a treatment option. During liver transplantation surgery the diseased liver is removed and a new healthy liver from a deceased-donor or a part of a liver from a living-donor is put in its place. Liver transplantation surgery is a major undertaking and requires life-long anti-rejection medications afterwards. Extensive testing is required before a liver transplant to ensure that a candidate is in good enough health to proceed with a transplant operation. Additionally, transplant centers typically require some period of abstinence from alcohol (often at least 6 months) and/or formal alcohol and drug treatment for patients with alcohol-related liver disease before transplantation. *Not all patients with cirrhosis need a liver transplant and transplantation is not the best choice for all patients.* Because liver transplantation is so complex it is only performed at large specialty centers and your doctor may need to refer you elsewhere in order to be evaluated for a liver transplant.

REVIEW QUESTIONS

ESSAY QUESTIONS

1. a. Classify the drugs used in treatment of asthma giving 2 examples for each class.
    b. Describe all the pharmacological actions of Ephedrine and salbutamol.
2. a. Explain briefly the terms hepatitis, Cirrhosis, Ulcerative colitis.
    b. Write short notes on Hepatitis.
3. Illustriate the drugs used in the treatment of ulcerative colitis.
4. Describe various GI disorders, Illustraite the therapeutic management of Peptic Ulcers and Ulcerative Colitis.
5. Write in detail on a) Enteric infections   b) Urinary tract infections.
6. Write in brief Epidemology, pathogenesis, investigation and treatment of Peptic Ulcer.

SHORT ANSWER QUESTIONS

7. Describe various GI disorders.
8. Write in detail on Urinary tract infections.
9. Write short notes on Hepatitis.
10. Classify the drugs used in treatment of asthma.
11. Write a short note on Cirrhosis.

Chapter 5

ENDOCRINE DISORDERS

5.1 DIABETES MELLITUS

Diabetes mellitus, often simply referred to as **diabetes** - is a group of metabolic diseases in which a person has high <u>blood sugar</u>, either because the body does not produce enough <u>insulin</u>, or because cells do not respond to the insulin that is produced. This high blood sugar produces the classical symptoms of <u>polyuria</u> (frequent urination), <u>polydipsia</u> (increased thirst) and <u>polyphagia</u> (increased hunger).

There are three main types of diabetes:

- **Type 1 diabetes**: results from the body's failure to produce insulin, and presently requires the person to inject insulin. (Also referred to as *insulin-dependent* diabetes mellitus, *IDDM* for short, and *juvenile* diabetes.)

- **Type 2 diabetes**: results from <u>insulin resistance</u>, a condition in which cells fail to use insulin properly, sometimes combined with an absolute insulin deficiency.

- **Gestational diabetes**: is when pregnant women, who have never had diabetes before, have a high blood glucose level during pregnancy. It may precede development of type 2 DM.

The term *diabetes*, without qualification, usually refers to diabetes mellitus, which roughly translates to excessive sweet urine (known as "<u>glycosuria</u>"). Several rare conditions are also named diabetes. The most common of these is <u>diabetes insipidus</u> in which large amounts of urine are produced (polyuria), which is not sweet (insipidus meaning "without taste" in Latin).

The term "type 1 diabetes" has replaced several former terms, including childhood-onset diabetes, juvenile diabetes, and insulin-dependent diabetes mellitus (IDDM). Likewise, the term "type 2 diabetes" has replaced several former terms, including adult-onset diabetes, obesity-related diabetes, and non-insulin-dependent diabetes mellitus (NIDDM). Beyond these two types, there is no agreed-upon standard nomenclature. Various sources have defined "type 3 diabetes" as: gestational diabetes, insulin-resistant type 1 diabetes (or "double diabetes"), type 2 diabetes which has progressed to require injected insulin, and latent autoimmune diabetes of adults (or LADA or "type 1.5" diabetes).

PRE-DIABETES

In pre-diabetes, blood glucose levels are higher than normal but not high enough for a diagnosis of diabetes. However, many people with pre-diabetes develop type 2 diabetes within 10 years. Experts disagree about the specific blood glucose level they should use to diagnose diabetes, and through the years, that number has changed. Individuals with pre-diabetes have an increased risk of heart disease and stroke. With modest weight loss and moderate physical activity, people with pre-diabetes can delay or prevent type 2 diabetes.

CLASSIFICATION

Most cases of diabetes mellitus fall into three broad categories: type 1, type 2, and gestational diabetes. A few other types are described.

TYPE 1 DIABETES

Type 1 diabetes mellitus is characterized by loss of the insulin-producing beta cells of the islets of Langerhans in the pancreas leading to insulin deficiency. This type of diabetes can be further classified as immune-mediated or idiopathic. The majority of type 1 diabetes is of the immune-mediated nature, where beta cell loss is a T-cell mediated autoimmune attack. There is no known preventive measure against type 1 diabetes, which causes approximately 10% of diabetes mellitus cases in North America and Europe. Most affected people are otherwise healthy and of a healthy weight when onset occurs. Sensitivity and responsiveness to insulin are usually normal, especially in the early stages. Type 1 diabetes can affect children or adults but was traditionally termed "juvenile diabetes" because it represents a majority of the diabetes cases in children.

TYPE 2 DIABETES

Type 2 diabetes mellitus is characterized by insulin resistance which may be combined with relatively reduced insulin secretion. The defective responsiveness of body tissues to insulin is believed to involve the insulin receptor. However, the specific defects are not known. Diabetes mellitus due to a known defect are classified separately. Type 2 diabetes is the most common type.

In the early stage of type 2 diabetes, the predominant abnormality is reduced insulin sensitivity. At this stage hyperglycemia can be reversed by a variety of measures and medications that improve insulin sensitivity or reduce glucose production by the liver.

GESTATIONAL DIABETES

Gestational diabetes mellitus (GDM) resembles type 2 diabetes in several respects, involving a combination of relatively inadequate insulin secretion and responsiveness. It occurs in about 2%–5% of all pregnancies and may improve or disappear after delivery. Gestational diabetes is fully treatable but requires careful medical supervision throughout the pregnancy. About 20%–50% of affected women develop type 2 diabetes later in life.

Even though it may be transient, untreated gestational diabetes can damage the health of the fetus or mother. Risks to the baby include macrosomia (high birth weight), congenital cardiac and central nervous system anomalies, and skeletal muscle malformations. Increased fetal insulin may inhibit fetal surfactant production and cause respiratory distress syndrome. Hyperbilirubinemia may result from red blood cell destruction. In severe cases, perinatal death may occur, most commonly as a result of poor placental perfusion due to vascular impairment. Labor induction may be indicated with decreased placental function. A cesarean section may be performed if there is marked fetal distress or an increased risk of injury associated with macrosomia, such as shoulder dystocia.

OTHER TYPES

Pre-diabetes indicates a condition that occurs when a person's blood glucose levels are higher than normal but not high enough for a diagnosis of type 2 diabetes. Many people destined to develop type 2 diabetes spend many years in a state of pre-diabetes which has been termed "America's largest healthcare epidemic."

Some cases of diabetes are caused by the body's tissue receptors not responding to insulin (even when insulin levels are normal, which is what separates it from type 2 diabetes); this form is very uncommon. Genetic mutations (autosomal or mitochondrial) can lead to defects in beta cell function. Abnormal insulin action may also have been genetically determined in some cases. Any disease that causes extensive damage to the pancreas may lead to diabetes (for example, chronic pancreatitis and cystic fibrosis). Diseases associated with excessive secretion of insulin-antagonistic hormones can cause diabetes (which is typically resolved once the hormone excess is removed).

Following is a comprehensive list of other causes of diabetes:

➢ Genetic defects of a-cell Function • Maturity onset diabetes of the young (MODY) • Mitochondrial DNA mutations ➢ Genetic defects in insulin processing or insulin action • Defects in proinsulin conversion • Insulin gene mutations • Insulin receptor mutations ➢ Exocrine Pancreatic Defects • Chronic pancreatitis • Pancreatectomy • Pancreatic neoplasia • Cystic fibrosis • Hemochromatosis • Fibrocalculous • pancreatopathy	➢ Endocrinopathies • Growth hormone excess (acromegaly) • Cushing syndrome • Hyperthyroidism • Pheochromocytoma • Glucagonoma ➢ Infections • Cytomegalovirus infection • Coxsackievirus B ➢ Drugs • Glucocorticoids • Thyroid hormone • β-adrenergic agonists

SIGNS AND SYMPTOMS

The classical symptoms of diabetes are polyuria (frequent urination), polydipsia (increased thirst) and polyphagia (increased hunger). Symptoms may develop rapidly (weeks or months) in type 1 diabetes while in type 2 diabetes they usually develop much more slowly and may be subtle or absent.

Prolonged high blood glucose causes glucose absorption, which leads to changes in the shape of the lenses of the eyes, resulting in vision changes; sustained sensible glucose control usually returns the lens to its original shape. Blurred vision is a common complaint leading to a diabetes diagnosis; type 1 should always be suspected in cases of rapid vision change, whereas with type 2 change is generally more gradual, but should still be suspected.

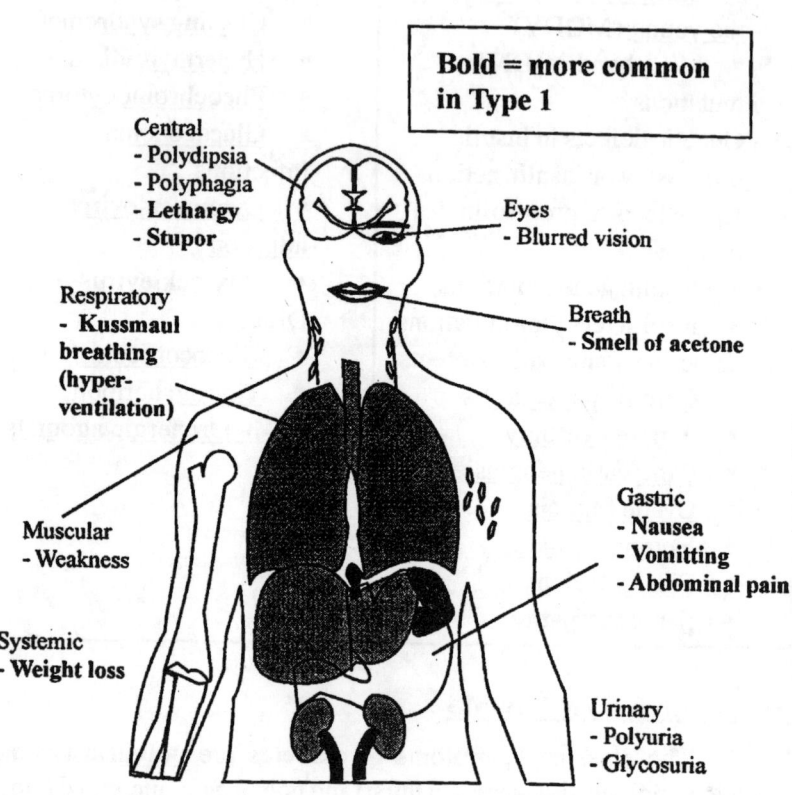

Fig .1. Overview of the most significant symptoms of diabetes

People (usually with type 1 diabetes) may also present with <u>diabetic ketoacidosis,</u> a state of metabolic dysregulation characterized by the smell of <u>acetone;</u> a rapid, deep breathing known as <u>Kussmaul breathing;</u> nausea; vomiting and <u>abdominal pain;</u> and an altered states of consciousness.

A rarer but equally severe possibility is <u>hyperosmolar nonketotic state</u>, which is more common in type 2 diabetes and is mainly the result of dehydration. Often, the patient has been drinking extreme amounts of sugar-containing drinks, leading to a <u>vicious circle</u> in regard to the water loss.

A number of skin rashes can occur in diabetes that are collectively known as <u>diabetic dermadromes</u>.

CAUSES OF DIABETES

Diabetes mellitus occurs when the pancreas doesn't make enough or any of the hormone insulin, or when the insulin produced doesn't work effectively. In diabetes, this causes the level of glucose in the blood to be too high.

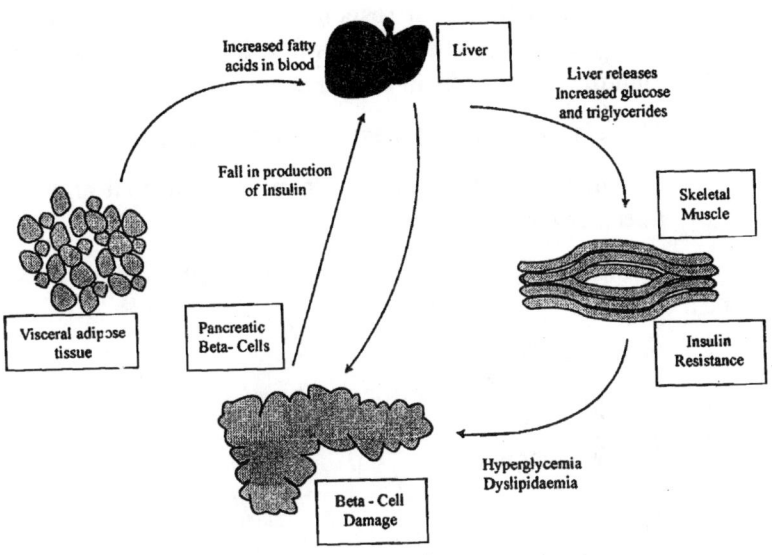

Fig.2. Major cause of Diabetes

In **Type 1 diabetes** the cells in the pancreas that make insulin are destroyed, causing a severe lack of insulin. This is thought to be the result of the body attacking and destroying its own cells in the pancreas - known as an autoimmune reaction.

It's not clear why this happens, but a number of explanations and possible triggers of this reaction have been proposed. These include:

- Infection with a specific virus or bacteria;

- Exposure to food-borne chemical toxins; and

- Exposure as a very young infant to cow's milk, where an as yet unidentified component of this triggers the autoimmune reaction in the body.

However, these are only hypotheses and are by no means proven causes.

Type 2 diabetes is believed to develop when:

- The receptors on cells in the body that normally respond to the action of insulin fail to be stimulated by it - this is known as insulin resistance. In response to this more insulin may be produced, and this over-production exhausts the insulin-manufacturing cells in the pancreas;

- There is simply insufficient insulin available; and

- The insulin that is available may be abnormal and therefore doesn't work properly.

The following risk factors increase the chances of someone developing Type 2 diabetes:

- Increasing age;

- Obesity; and

- Physical inactivity.

Rarer causes of diabetes include:

- Certain medicines;

- Pregnancy (gestational diabetes); and

- Any illness or disease that damages the pancreas and affects its ability to produce insulin e.g. pancreatitis.

DIAGNOSIS OF DIABETES

The following tests are used for diagnosis:

- A **fasting plasma glucose (FPG) test** measures blood glucose in a person who has not eaten anything for at least 8 hours. This test is used to detect diabetes and pre-diabetes.

- An **oral glucose tolerance test (OGTT)** measures blood glucose after a person fasts at least 8 hours and 2 hours after the person drinks a glucose-containing beverage. This test can be used to diagnose diabetes and pre-diabetes.

- A **random plasma glucose test**, also called a casual plasma glucose test, measures blood glucose without regard to when the person being tested last ate. This test, along with an assessment of symptoms, is used to diagnose diabetes but not pre-diabetes.

Test results indicating that a person has diabetes should be confirmed with a second test on a different day.

FPG TEST

Table 1. FPG test

Plasma Glucose Result (mg/dL)	Diagnosis
99 or below	Normal
100 to 125	Pre-diabetes (impaired fasting glucose)
126 or above	Diabetes

The FPG test is the preferred test for diagnosing diabetes because of its convenience and low cost. However, it will miss some diabetes or pre-diabetes that can be found with the OGTT. The FPG test is most reliable when done in the morning. Results and their meaning are shown in Table 1. People with a fasting glucose level of 100 to 125 milligrams per deciliter (mg/dL) have a form of pre-diabetes called impaired fasting glucose (IFG). Having IFG means a person has an increased risk of developing type 2 diabetes but does not have it yet. A level of 126 mg/dL or above, confirmed by repeating the test on another day, means a person has diabetes.

OGTT

Research has shown that the OGTT is more sensitive than the FPG test for diagnosing pre-diabetes, but it is less convenient to administer. The OGTT requires fasting for at least 8 hours before the test. The plasma glucose level is measured immediately before and 2 hours after a person drinks a liquid containing 75 grams of glucose dissolved in water. Results and their meaning are shown in Table 2. If the blood glucose level is between 140 and 199 mg/dL 2 hours after drinking the liquid, the person has a form of pre-diabetes called impaired glucose tolerance (IGT). Having IGT, like having IFG, means a person has an increased risk of developing type 2 diabetes but does not have it yet. A 2-hour glucose level of 200 mg/dL or above, confirmed by repeating the test on another day, means a person has diabetes.

Table 2. OGTT

2-hour Plasma Glucose Result (mg/dL)	Diagnosis
139 or below	Normal
140 to 199	Pre-diabetes (impaired glucose tolerance)
200 or above	Diabetes

Gestational diabetes is also diagnosed based on plasma glucose values measured during the OGTT, preferably by using 100 grams of glucose in liquid for the test. Blood glucose levels are checked four times during the test. If blood glucose levels are above normal at least twice during the test, the woman has gestational diabetes. Table 3 shows the above-normal results for the OGTT for gestational diabetes.

Table 3. Gestational diabetes: Above-normal results for the OGTT

When	Plasma Glucose Result (mg/dL)
Fasting	95 or higher
At 1 hours	180 or higher
At 2 hours	155 or higher
At 3 hours	140 or higher

Random Plasma Glucose Test

A random, or casual, blood glucose level of 200 mg/dL or higher, plus the presence of the following symptoms, can mean a person has diabetes:

- Increased urination
- Increased thirst
- Unexplained weight loss

Other symptoms can include fatigue, blurred vision, increased hunger, and sores that do not heal. The doctor will check the person's blood glucose level on another day using the FPG test or the OGTT to confirm the diagnosis.

TREATMENT OF DIABETES

The goal of treatment for diabetes is to maintain blood glucose levels as close to normal as possible. There are three basic treatments:

I.   **Diet:** Changes in diet to be 30% fat (mostly monounsaturated fat and polyunsaturated), 40-55% carbohydrates (high fiber, low glycemic index) and 15% protein. The distribution of carbohydrates and calories throughout the day are important, as well as limiting total calories to achieve a near ideal body weight. These changes will lower blood glucose and lipid levels.

II.   Exercise: Exercise burns calories and muscle glycogen, which lowers blood glucose. Exercise decreases insulin resistance, which allows insulin to normally manage glucose levels.

III.   Medications:

a.   Oral medications reduce blood glucose levels by improving insulin release from the pancreas, reducing the available glucose or decreasing insulin resistance.

b.   Injectable medications:

Insulin is injected to replace the insulin the body can no longer produce. Insulin reduces blood glucose.

Exenatide (brand name Byetta) is an incretin mimetic that mimics a hormone that creates more insulin. Also acts as an appetite suppressant.

Pramlintide is a synthetic form of a hormone amylin, which is limited in the person with diabetes. Amylin slows the emptying of the stomach and regulates the rate of blood glucose rise.

Diet and exercise are the basis of treatment. Medication - oral medicine or injected insulin and other agents - are added if blood glucose goal are not achieved.

MEDICAL TREATMENT

The treatment of diabetes is highly individualized, depending on the type of diabetes, whether the patient has other active medical problems, whether the patient has complications of diabetes, and age and general health of the patient at time of diagnosis.

- A healthcare provider will set goals for lifestyle changes, blood sugar control, and treatment.

- Together, the patient and the healthcare provider will devise a plan to help meet those goals.

Education about diabetes and its treatment is essential in all types of diabetes.

- When the patient is first diagnosed with diabetes, the diabetes care team will spend a lot of time with the patient, teaching them about their condition, treatment, and everything they need to know to care for themselves on a daily basis.

- The diabetes care team includes the healthcare provider and his or her staff. It may include specialists in foot care, neurology, kidney diseases, and eye diseases. A professional dietitian and a diabetes educator also may be part of the team.

The healthcare team will see you at appropriate intervals to monitor your progress with your goals.

TYPE 1 DIABETES

Treatment of diabetes almost always involves the daily injection of insulin, usually a combination of short-acting insulin [for example, lispro (Humalog) or aspart (NovoLog)] and longer acting insulin [for example, NPH, Lente, glargine (Lantus), detemir, or ultralente].

- Insulin must be given as an injection. If taken by mouth, insulin would be destroyed in the stomach before it could get into the blood where it is needed.

- Most people with type 1 diabetes give these injections to themselves. Even if someone else usually gives the patient injections, it is important that the patient knows how to do it in case the other person is unavailable.

- A trained professional will show the patient how to store and inject the insulin. Usually this is a nurse who works with the healthcare provider or a diabetes educator.

- Insulin is usually given in two or three injections per day, generally around mealtimes. Dosage is individualized and is tailored to the patient's specific needs by the healthcare provider. Longer acting insulins are typically administered one or two times per day.

- Some people have their insulin administered by continuous infusion pumps to provide adequate blood glucose control. Supplemental mealtime insulin is programmed into the pump by the individual as recommended by his or her healthcare provider.

- It is very important to eat if the patient has taken insulin, as the insulin will lower blood sugar regardless of whether they have eaten. If insulin is taken without eating, the result may be hypoglycemia. This is called an insulin reaction.

- There is an adjustment period while the patient learns how insulin affects them, and how to time meals and exercise with insulin injections to keep blood sugar level as even as possible.

- Keeping accurate records of blood sugar levels and insulin dosages is crucial for the patient's diabetes management.

- Eating a consistent, healthy diet appropriate for the patient's size and weight is essential in controlling blood sugar level.

TYPE 2 DIABETES

Depending on how elevated the patient's blood sugar and glycosylated hemoglobin (HbA1c) are at the time of diagnosis, they may be given a chance to lower blood sugar level without medication.

- The best way to do this is to lose weight if obese and begin an exercise program.

- This will generally be tried for three to six months, then blood sugar and glycosylated hemoglobin will be rechecked. If they remain high, the patient will be started on an oral medication, usually a sulfonylurea or biguanide [Metformin Glucophage], to help control blood sugar level.

- Even if the patient is on medication, it is still important to eat a healthy diet, lose weight if they are overweight, and engage in moderate physical activity as often as possible.

- The healthcare provider will monitor the patient's progress on medication very carefully at first. It is important to get just the right dose of the right medication to get the blood sugar level in the recommended range with the fewest side effects.

- The doctor may decide to combine two types of medications to get blood sugar level under control.

- Gradually, even people with type 2 diabetes may require insulin injections to control their blood sugar levels.

- It is becoming more common for people with type 2 diabetes to take a combination of oral medication and insulin injections to control blood sugar levels.

5.2 THYROID DISORDERS

Hormonal disorders or endocrine disorders, including thyroid disorders, are illnesses that occur when the body releases too many or too few hormones. Hormones are chemicals messengers that are released into the bloodstream. Hormones send messages to cells throughout the body in order to regulate bodily functions, such as growth, metabolism, and sexual development. As a result, individuals with hormonal disorders experience a disruption in such bodily functions.

Thyroid disorders are among the most common medical conditions but, because their symptoms often appear gradually over time, they are commonly misdiagnosed. There are four main types of thyroid disease: hyperthyroidism or too much thyroid hormone; hypothyroidism or too little thyroid hormone; benign (non-cancerous) thyroid disease; and thyroid cancer.

The thyroid gland is a small, butterfly-shaped gland located in the base of the neck on both sides of the lower part of the voice box (larynx) and upper part of the wind pipe (trachea). The thyroid produces hormones, called thyroxine (T4) and triiodothyronine (T3), which affect the body's metabolism and energy level. Thyroid hormone is also produced in response to thyroid stimulating hormone (TSH, also known as thyrotropin) secreted by the pituitary gland.

Release of thyroid hormones is controlled by the hypothalamus and pituitary gland, both found deep inside the brain. One of the most important features of the endocrine system is its regulation (control) by negative feedback. This means that the glands that stimulate the release of a hormone (for example, the pituitary) from another gland (for example, the thyroid) are eventually shut off, in a sense, so that too much hormone is not produced.

TYPES OF THYROID DISORDERS

Hyperthyroidism: Hyperthyroidism occurs when the thyroid gland produces too much thyroxine. As a result, the individual's metabolism increases dramatically, leading to weight loss and irregular heartbeat.

Most individuals fully recover from hyperthyroidism with treatment. However, if left untreated, the condition may be life threatening. Complications may include heart problems, brittle bones, and **thyrotoxic crisis** (sudden release of thyroid hormone). Thyrotoxic crisis occurs when symptoms suddenly become extreme, causing fever, increased heartbeat, and sometimes delirium.

The most common cause of hyperthyroidism is Grave's disease. In **Graves' disease,** a malfunction in the body's immune system releases abnormal antibodies that mimic thyroid stimulating hormone (TSH). Spurred by these false signals to produce, the thyroid's hormone factories work overtime and produce an excess of thyroid hormone.

Exophthalmia: also known as exophthalmos is bulging of the eyes. Exophthalmia is a characteristic of individuals with Grave's disease. Exophthalmia occurs in about 40-60% of individuals who suffer from Grave's disease.

Non-cancerous tumors (abnormal growths) on the thyroid gland may also lead to hyperthyroidism. Some tumors may cause the thyroid to produce excess thyroid hormone. This causes the thyroid to become enlarged.

Hyperthyroidism may also occur if the thyroid gland becomes inflamed, called **thyroiditis**. When the gland is swollen, stored thyroid hormone may leak into the bloodstream.

Hypothyroidism: Hypothyroidism occurs when the thyroid gland does not produce enough thyroid hormone.

A condition called **Hashimoto's thyroiditis** is the most common cause of hypothyroidism in the United States. Thyroiditis is an inflammation of the thyroid gland not due to infection. Several types of thyroiditis exist and the treatment is different for each. Hashimoto's thyroiditis occurs when the individual's immune system attacks the thyroid gland, causing low levels of thyroid hormone. Researchers have not discovered why the immune system mistakes the thyroid for a harmful invader, such as a virus. It has been suggested that many factors lead to the disorder, including age, heredity, and gender. This is because the condition is most common among middle-aged women. It is also common among biological family members.

Other less common types of hypothyroidism include De Quervain's thyroiditis and silent thyroiditis. In De Quervain's thyroiditis the thyroid gland generally swells rapidly and is very painful and tender. In silent thyroiditis, there is no pain or needle biopsy (removal of tissue for examination).

Hypothyroidism may also occur if individuals do not consume enough iodine in the diet. This is most common in poor countries where malnutrition is common. Iodine is an essential element that helps the thyroid gland produce hormones.

A goiter is an enlargement of the thyroid gland. Although generally not uncomfortable, goiter can interfere with swallowing or breathing. Goiters are more common in women and older adults. The most common cause of goiter is a shortage of iodine in the diet in areas where the soil is deficient in iodine. Although goiters generally do not cause pain, a large goiter may interfere with swallowing or breathing and it may affect the individual's appearance and self-esteem. In many cases, goiters will be cured once hormone replacement therapy is started. However, some individuals may need to have their goiter surgically removed. Goiters are typical of hypothyroidism.

Individuals should visit their healthcare providers every six to 12 months to monitor their hormone levels. Over time, the dosage of thyroid medication may need to be changed. If the dose is too high, individuals may develop a condition called osteoporosis, which causes the bones to become hollow and brittle. Also, excessive doses may lead to irregular heartbeats (arrhythmias). In order to prevent complications of overdose, individuals with a history of heart disease, osteoporosis, or severe hypothyroidism may receive smaller doses that are gradually increased over time.

Thyroid nodules: Thyroid nodules are lumps that commonly arise within an otherwise normal thyroid gland. Often these abnormal growths of thyroid tissue are located at the edge of the thyroid gland so they can be felt as a lump in the throat. When they are large or when they occur in very thin individuals, they can even sometimes be seen as a lump in the front of the neck. One in 12-15 young women has a thyroid nodule, and one in 40 young men have a thyroid nodule. More than 95% of all thyroid nodules are benign (non-cancerous growths). Some nodules are actually cysts that are filled with fluid rather than thyroid tissue. Most individuals will develop a thyroid nodule by the time they are 50 years old. The incidence of thyroid nodules increases with age; 50% of 50 year olds will have at least one thyroid nodule, 60% of 60 year olds will have at least one thyroid nodule, and 70% of 70 year olds will have at least one thyroid nodule. Individuals do not have to have hypo- and hyperthyroidism to have nodules of the thyroid gland.

Thyroid cancer: Many types of tumors can develop in the thyroid gland. Most of these tumors are benign (non-cancerous). Others are malignant (cancerous), which means they can spread into nearby tissues and to other parts of the body. Anyone can get cancer of the thyroid gland, but certain factors may increase the risk. Risk factors include: being between ages 25-65; being a woman; being Asian; having a family member who has had thyroid disease; or having radiation treatments to the head or neck.

Hyperparathyroidism: The parathyroid glands regulate serum calcium and phosphorus levels through the secretion of parathyroid hormone (PTH), which raises serum calcium levels while lowering the serum phosphorus concentration. The regulation of PTH secretion occurs through a negative feedback loop in which calcium-sensing receptors on the membranes of parathyroid cells trigger decreased PTH production as serum calcium concentrations rise. Primary hyperparathyroidism, which accounts for most presentations of hyperparathyroidism, results from excessive release of PTH and manifests as hypercalcemia. In 80% of patients with hyperparathyroidism, the symptoms of hypercalcemia (high blood levels of calcium) are mild or not notable.

Hypoparathyroidism: Hypoparathyroidism is secretion of too little parathyroid hormone. The symptoms of hypoparathyroidism are the same as hypocalcemia (low blood calcium levels). Symptoms can range from quite mild (tingling in the hands, fingers, and around the mouth) to more severe forms of muscle cramps leading all the way to tetany (severe muscle cramping of the entire body), and rarely convulsions.

CAUSES AND RISK FACTORS

Risk factors for developing thyroid disorders include: previous thyroid dysfunction; goiter; surgery or radiotherapy affecting the thyroid gland; diabetes mellitus; vitiligo, an autoimmune disorder in which white patches of skin appear on different parts of the body; pernicious anemia, or a condition where red blood cells are not providing adequate oxygen to body tissues; leukotrichia (prematurely gray hair); adrenal insufficiency; and medications and other compounds, such as lithium carbonate and iodine-containing compounds, such as amiodarone hydrochloride, radio contrast agents, expectorants containing potassium iodide, and kelp. A lack of vitamin B12 may put an individual at risk for developing a thyroid condition.

Hypothyroidism: The causes of hypothyroidism include: heredity; Hashimoto's disease; pituitary tumors; thyroiditis (inflammation of the thyroid gland caused by excessive amounts of thyroid hormone leaking out of the thyroid gland and into the blood); not enough thyroid hormone medication; surgical removal of thyroid tissue (thyroidectomy); radioactive iodine administration; and a dietary deficiency of iodine.

Hyperthyroidism: The causes of hyperthyroidism include: heredity; Grave's disease, also known as toxic diffuse goiter (enlargement of the thyroid gland); Plummer's disease, a condition where there is a single nodule (called adenoma) producing excess thyroid hormone; pituitary tumors; thyroiditis (inflammation of the thyroid gland caused by excessive amounts of thyroid hormone leaking out of the thyroid gland and into the blood); too much thyroid hormone medication; and excessive dietary intake of iodine (found in seaweed and liver).

SIGNS AND SYMPTOMS

Hypothyroidism: Common symptoms of hypothyroidism include sensitivity to cold temperatures, mild weight gain, fatigue, constipation, small thyroid gland, enlarged neck, dry skin, hair loss, muscle cramps, heavy and irregular menstruation, and difficulty thinking or concentrating. Less common symptoms main include facial swelling and joint stiffness. The most obvious sign of severe hypothyroidism is a goiter. A goiter is a severe swelling of the thyroid gland in the front of the neck.

Hyperthyroidism: Common symptoms of hyperthyroidism include sudden and unexplained weight loss, increased or irregular heartbeat, nervousness, irritability, tremors (especially in the hands), increased sweating, abnormal menstruation, increased sensitivity to warmth, more frequent bowel movements, enlarged thyroid gland (goiter), fatigue, difficulty sleeping, and muscle weakness. Some patients may be unable to close the eyelid (eyelid retraction). Some individuals may also experience lid-lag. This occurs when the eyelids do not move down when the person's eye looks downward.

DIAGNOSIS

Blood tests: A blood test that measures the amount of thyroid hormones in the blood is the standard diagnostic test for an underactive thyroid. If the individual has low levels of thyroid hormone in the blood, the patient is diagnosed with hypothyroidism.

The levels of thyroxine (T4), triiodothyronine (T3), and thyroid stimulating hormone (TSH) in the blood stream are measured. An overactive thyroid, such as in hyperthyroidism, would be expected to cause high levels of T4 and T3 and low levels of TSH. An underactive thyroid, such as in hypothyroidism, would be expected to cause low levels of T4 and T3 and a high level of TSH.

Subclinical hypothyroidism and hyperthyroidism: Some patients are found to have elevated serum thyroid stimulating hormone (TSH) levels, suggesting hypothyroidism, but have normal levels of thyroxine (T4). This state is referred to as subclinical hypothyroidism. Some individuals with subclinical hypothyroidism may have clinical symptoms, such as weakness, lethargy, fatigue, hoarseness, hearing loss, bradycardia (slow heart rate), dry skin, coarse hair, cold intolerance, constipation, weight gain, muscle cramps, and fluid build-up in the eyelids, face, and legs. Treatment of subclinical hypothyroidism is similar to hypothyroidism.

Subclinical hyperthyroidism is defined as low serum TSH concentrations in the presence of normal serum thyroid hormone concentrations (T4 or FT4 and T3 or FT3 levels). Individuals with subclinical hyperthyroidism are at increased risk for cardiac arrhythmias and bone loss.

Fluorescent antinuclear antibody (FANA) test: The fluorescent antinuclear antibody (FANA) test may be performed to detect abnormal antibodies, called auto antibodies. The auto antibodies bind to components of an individual's own cells and cause the immune system to attack the body. Antibodies are part of the body's immune system defense against foreign substances, such as bacteria and viruses.

During the procedure, a small sample of blood is taken from the individual and sent to a laboratory. A scientist adds methyl alcohol to a microscope slide that contains human tissue culture cells. This makes the cells permeable before they are combined with the individual's blood.

Then the individual's blood is added to the microscope slide. Fluorescent antibodies that detect the binding of human antibodies to the cells are also added. The scientist uses a fluorescent microscope to view the staining intensity and binding pattern of the cells. If auto antibodies are detected, a positive diagnosis is made for an autoimmune disorder.

If an individual has a positive FANA result and has low levels of thyroid hormone in the blood, Hashimoto's thyroiditis is diagnosed.

Ultrasound: Ultrasound takes a picture of the inside of the thyroid. Ultrasound bounces sound waves off the thyroid and makes a picture out of the returning echoes. If the ultrasound shows a large mass that is suspicious for cancer, then the doctor can use the ultrasound to guide a needle into the mass to perform a fine needle aspiration biopsy. If there are no large lumps in the thyroid gland that are suspicious for cancer, then no biopsy needs to be done.

Nuclear scan: Sometimes a nuclear medicine thyroid scan is ordered to help determine the cause of an individual's overactive thyroid. Individuals swallow capsules that contain a harmless radioactive tracer bound to iodine. Some of this tracer winds up in the thyroid gland. Four, six, or 24 hours after the capsule is ingested (depending on the preferences of the radiology department performing the scan), a scanner is placed over the thyroid gland. This scanner can take a picture of the thyroid gland by detecting the parts of the thyroid gland that have taken up the radioactive tracer.

In a normal thyroid gland, radioactive iodine is taken up to the same degree throughout the entire gland. If there is an area of the thyroid that does not take up radioactive iodine well, then it must be further investigated. It can be useful to measure how much of the radioactive tracer wound up in the thyroid gland. This can help determine the cause of the overactive thyroid. However, the actual diagnosis of the overactive thyroid is made with blood tests, not with the scan.

Biopsy: Thyroid nodules are fairly common and usually harmless. However, about 4% of nodules are cancerous, so further testing needs to be done. This is usually best accomplished by fine needle aspiration biopsy. This is a quick and simple test that takes just a few minutes to perform in the doctor's office. If the biopsy does not raise any suspicion of cancer, the nodule is usually observed over time to watch for any changes. Some thyroid specialists recommend treatment with thyroid hormone to try to decrease the size of the nodule. A second biopsy is usually recommended six to 12 months later, to make sure there continues to be no evidence of cancer. If a nodule is cancerous, suspicious for cancer, or grows large enough to interfere with swallowing or breathing, surgical removal is advised.

TREATMENT

Hypothyroidism:

General: Once individuals are diagnosed with hypothyroidism (underactive thyroid) or Hashimoto's thyroiditis, they receive man-made hormones to make up for the decreased hormone levels. Treatment is life-long. Some individuals may need to have their thyroid gland surgically removed. These people will need to take hormones for the rest of their lives, but they are able to live normal, healthy lives.

Individuals should tell their healthcare providers if they are taking any other drugs (prescription or over-the-counter), herbs, or supplements because they may interact with treatment. For instance, a cholesterol lowering medication called cholestyramine (Questran®), an ingredient in some antacids called aluminum hydroxide, sodium polystyrene sulfonate (Kayexalate®), an anti-ulcer drug called sucralfate (Carafate®), iron supplements, calcium supplements, and soy may interact with treatment.

Thyroid hormone replacement therapy: Individuals receive thyroid hormone replacement therapy with levothyroxine (Levothroid®, Levoxyl®, Synthroid®, or Unithroid®). This man-made hormone is identical to the natural thyroid hormone called thyroxine. The medication is taken by mouth every day for life to help the body return to normal functioning. A synthetic form of thyroid hormone, liothyronine (Cytomel®), may also be prescribed.

Individuals should visit their healthcare providers every six to 12 months to monitor their hormone levels. Over time, the dosage may be changed. If the dose is too high, individuals may develop a condition called osteoporosis, which causes the bones to become hollow and brittle. Also, excessive doses may lead to irregular heartbeats (arrhythmias). In order to prevent complications of overdose, individuals with a history of heart disease, osteoporosis, or severe hypothyroidism may receive smaller doses that are gradually increased over time.

Surgery: If an individual patient develops a goiter that does not respond to hormone therapy, the thyroid may need to be surgically removed (called thyroidectomy). Although goiters generally do not cause pain, a large goiter can interfere with swallowing or breathing and it may affect the individual's appearance and self-esteem. Individuals can live long, healthy lives without the thyroid gland. However, they must take hormone pills called levothyroxine (Levothroid®, Levoxyl®, Synthroid® or Unithroid®) for the rest of their lives.

Hyperthyroidism:

Several treatments for hyperthyroidism exist. The best approach depends on age, physical health, and the severity of the condition.

Radioactive iodine: Taken by mouth, radioactive iodine is absorbed by the thyroid gland, where it causes the gland to shrink and symptoms to subside, usually within three to six months. Because this treatment causes thyroid activity to slow considerably and for the thyroid gland to shrink in size, individuals may eventually need to take a medication every day to achieve adequate thyroid hormone levels.

Anti-thyroid medications: Anti-thyroid medications gradually reduce symptoms of hyperthyroidism by preventing the thyroid gland from producing excess amounts of hormones. They include propylthiouracil (PTU) and methimazole (Tapazole®). Symptoms usually begin to improve in six to 12 weeks, but treatment with anti-thyroid medications typically continues at least a year and often longer. For some individuals, symptoms of hyperthyroidism disappear completely, but others may experience a relapse.

Beta blockers: Beta blockers are commonly used to treat hypertension (high blood pressure). They will not reduce thyroid levels, but they can reduce a rapid heart rate and help prevent palpitations. Individuals with hyperthyroidism may be prescribed beta blockers until the thyroid levels are closer to normal and heart symptoms disappear.

Surgery: Thyroidectomy is used when the individual cannot tolerate anti-thyroid drugs and does not want to have radioactive iodine therapy, although this is an option in only a few cases. These individuals may be at an increased risk for complications when using drugs or radioactive therapy.

In a thyroidectomy, a doctor removes most of the thyroid gland. Risks of this surgery include damage to the vocal cords and parathyroid glands. Parathyroid glands are four tiny glands located on the back of the thyroid gland that help control the level of calcium in the blood. Individuals undergoing a thyroidectomy will need lifelong treatment with levothyroxine (Synthroid®) to supply the body with normal amounts of thyroid hormone. If the parathyroid glands also are removed, individuals will need medication to keep the blood-calcium levels normal.

PREVENTION

The American Thyroid Association recommends that adults be screened for thyroid dysfunction by measurement of the serum thyrotropin (also known as thyroid stimulating hormone or TSH) concentration beginning at age 35 years and every five years thereafter. Individuals with symptoms and signs potentially attributable to thyroid dysfunction and those with risk factors for its development may require more frequent serum thyrotropin testing.

Iodine deficiency is the most common cause of hypothyroidism worldwide. Iodine is found in seawater, so any type of seafood is a rich source of this element, particularly seaweed (including kelp, bladderwrack, or dulce). Despite coming from the ocean, sea salt is not a good source of iodine. Iodized salt is perhaps the most common source of iodine in the Western diet and can provide enough iodine to avoid low thyroid activity. Since an adult only requires around one teaspoonful of iodine over a lifetime, eating fish once a week is enough to fulfill the average iodine requirement.

The value of dietary iodine can be reduced by vegetables from the brassica family, which includes cabbage, brussels sprouts, raw turnip, broccoli, and cauliflower. In circumstances where both large quantities of these foods are eaten and the levels of dietary iodine are low, goiter could develop.

Exercise is important for maintaining healthy hormone levels. Exercise 30 minutes daily, five days a week if possible. A doctor can help design an exercise program that is right for each individual.

INFECTIOUS DISEASES

5.3 TUBERCULOSIS

Tuberculosis (TB) is an infectious disease caused by bacteria whose scientific name is _Mycobacterium tuberculosis_. It was first isolated in 1882 by a German physician named Robert Koch who received the Nobel Prize for this discovery. TB most commonly affects the lungs but also can involve almost any organ of the body. It is spread through the air when people who have the disease cough, sneeze, or spit. Most infections in humans result in an asymptomatic, latent infection, and about one in ten latent infections eventually progresses to active disease, which, if left untreated, kills more than 50% of its victims.

The classic symptoms are a chronic cough with blood-tinged sputum, fever, night sweats, and weight loss (the last giving rise to the formerly prevalent colloquial term "consumption"). Infection of other organs causes a wide range of symptoms. Diagnosis relies on radiology (commonly chest X-rays), a tuberculin skin test, blood tests, as well as microscopic examination and microbiological of bodily fluids. Treatment is difficult and requires long courses of multiple antibiotics. Contacts are also screened and treated if necessary. Antibiotic resistance is a growing problem in (extensively) multi-drug-resistant tuberculosis. Prevention relies on screening programs and vaccination, usually with Bacillus Calmette-Guerin vaccine.

One third of the world's population is thought to be infected with *M. tuberculosis*, and new infections occur at a rate of about one per second. The proportion of people who become sick with tuberculosis each year is stable or falling worldwide but, because of population growth, the absolute number of new cases is still increasing. In 2007 there were an estimated 13.7 million chronic active cases, 9.3 million new cases, and 1.8 million deaths, mostly in developing countries. In addition, more people in the developed world are contracting tuberculosis because their immune systems are compromised by immunosuppressive drugs, substance abuse, or AIDS. The distribution of tuberculosis is not uniform across the globe; about 80% of the population in many Asian and African countries test positive in tuberculin tests, while only 5-10% of the US population test positive.

CLASSIFICATION

The current clinical classification system for tuberculosis (TB) is based on the pathogenesis of the disease.

Table 4. Classification System for TB

Class	Type	Description
0	No TB exposure Not infected	No history of exposure Negative reaction to tuberculin skin test
1	TB exposure No evidence of infection	History of exposure Negative reaction to tuberculin skin test Ghon complex
2	TB infection No disease	Positive reaction to tuberculin skin test Negative bacteriologic studies (if done) Fibrocaseous cavitary lesion (usually in upper lobe of lungs)
3	TB, clinically active	*M. tuberculosis* cultured (if done) Clinical, bacteriologic, or radiographic evidence of current disease
4	TB Not clinically active	History of episode(s) of TB or Abnormal but stable radiographic findings, Positive reaction to the tuberculin skin test Negative bacteriologic studies (if done) and No clinical or radiographic evidence of current disease
5	TB suspect	Diagnosis pending TB disease should be ruled in or out within 3 months

When the disease becomes active, 75% of the cases are pulmonary TB, that is, TB in the lungs. Symptoms include chest pain, coughing up blood, and a productive, prolonged cough for more than three weeks. Systemic symptoms include fever, chills, night sweats, appetite loss, weight loss, pallor, and often a tendency to fatigue very easily.

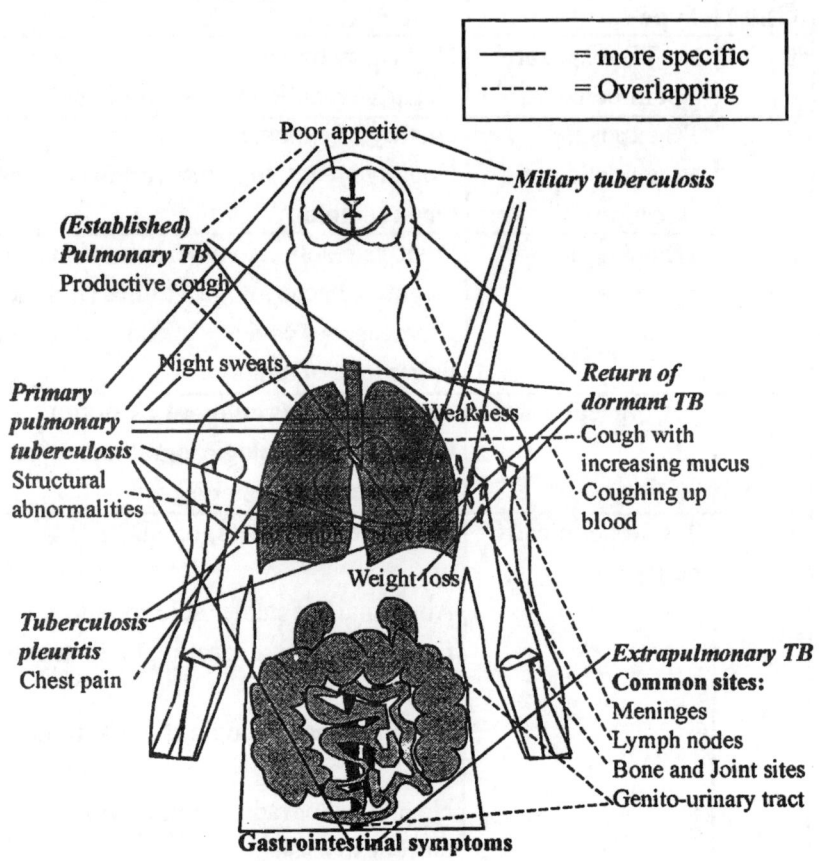

| —— | = more specific |
| ----- | = Overlapping |

Fig.3. Main Symptoms of Tuberculosis(TB)

In the other 25% of active cases, the infection moves from the lungs, causing other kinds of TB, collectively denoted extrapulmonary tuberculosis. This occurs more commonly in immunosuppressed persons and young children. Extrapulmonary infection sites include the pleura in tuberculosis pleurisy, the central nervous system in meningitis, the lymphatic system in scrofula of the neck, the genitourinary

system in urogenital tuberculosis, and bones and joints in Pott's disease of the spine. An especially serious form is disseminated TB, more commonly known as miliary tuberculosis. Extrapulmonary TB may co-exist with pulmonary TB as well.

TUBERCULOSIS CAUSES

All cases of TB are passed from person to person via droplets. When someone with TB infection coughs, sneezes, or talks, tiny droplets of saliva or mucus are expelled into the air, which can be inhaled by another person.

- Once infectious particles reach the alveoli (small saclike structures in the air spaces in the lungs), another cell, called the macrophage, engulfs the TB bacteria.

  o Then the bacteria are transmitted to the lymphatic system and bloodstream and spread to other organs occurs.

  o The bacteria further multiply in organs that have high oxygen pressures, such as the upper lobes of the lungs, the kidneys, bone marrow, and meninges the membrane-like coverings of the brain and spinal cord.

- When the bacteria cause clinically detectable disease, you have TB.

- People who have inhaled the TB bacteria, but in whom the disease is controlled, are referred to as infected. Their immune system has walled off the organism in an inflammatory focus known as a granuloma. They have no symptoms, frequently have a positive skin test for TB, yet cannot transmit the disease to others. This is referred to as latent tuberculosis infection or LTBI.

- Risk factors for TB include the following:

  o HIV infection,

  o Low socioeconomic status

  o Alcoholism

  o Homelessness,

o   Crowded living conditions,

o   Diseases that weaken the immune system,

o   Migration from a country with a high number of cases,

o   And health-care workers.

MECHANISM

Transmission

When people suffering from active pulmonary TB cough, sneeze, speak, or spit, they expel infectious aerosol droplets 0.5 to 5 μm in diameter. A single sneeze can release up to 40,000 droplets. Each one of these droplets may transmit the disease, since the infectious dose of tuberculosis is very low and inhaling less than ten bacteria may cause an infection.

People with prolonged, frequent, or intense contact are at particularly high risk of becoming infected, with an estimated 22% infection rate. A person with active but untreated tuberculosis can infect 10-15 other people per year. Others at risk include people in areas where TB is common, people who inject drugs using unsanitary needles, residents and employees of high-risk congregate settings, medically under-served and low-income populations, high-risk racial or ethnic minority populations, children exposed to adults in high-risk categories, patients immunocompromised by conditions such as HIV/AIDS, people who take immunosuppressant drugs, and health care workers serving these high-risk clients.

Transmission can only occur from people with active TB. The probability of transmission from one person to another depends upon the number of infectious droplets expelled by a carrier, the effectiveness of ventilation, the duration of exposure, and the virulence of the M. tuberculosis strain. The chain of transmission can, therefore, be broken by isolating patients with active disease and starting effective anti-tuberculous therapy. After two weeks of such treatment, people with non-resistant active TB generally cease to be contagious. If someone does become infected, then it will take at least 21 days, or three to four weeks, before the newly infected person can transmit the disease to others. TB can also be transmitted by eating meat infected with TB. *Mycobacterium bovis* causes TB in cattle.

Pathogenesis

About 90% of those infected with *Mycobacterium tuberculosis* have asymptomatic, latent TB infection (sometimes called LTBI), with only a 10% lifetime chance that a latent infection will progress to TB disease. However, if untreated, the death rate for these active TB cases is more than 50%.

TB infection begins when the mycobacteria reach the pulmonary alveoli, where they invade and replicate within the endosomes of alveolar macrophages. The primary site of infection in the lungs is called the Ghon focus, and is generally located in either the upper part of the lower lobe, or the lower part of the upper lobe. Bacteria are picked up by dendritic cells, which do not allow replication, although these cells can transport the bacilli to local (mediastinal) lymph nodes. Further spread is through the bloodstream to other tissues and organs where secondary TB lesions can develop in other parts of the lung (particularly the apex of the upper lobes), peripheral lymph nodes, kidneys, brain, and bone. All parts of the body can be affected by the disease, though it rarely affects the heart, skeletal muscles, pancreas and thyroid.

Tuberculosis is classified as one of the granulomatous inflammatory conditions. Macrophages, T lymphocytes, B lymphocytes and fibroblasts are among the cells that aggregate to form a granuloma, with lymphocytes surrounding the infected macrophages. The granuloma functions not only to prevent dissemination of the mycobacteria, but also provides a local environment for communication of cells of the immune system. Within the granuloma, T lymphocytes secrete cytokines such as interferon gamma, which activates macrophages to destroy the bacteria with which they are infected. Cytotoxic T cells can also directly kill infected cells, by secreting perforin and granulysin.

Importantly, bacteria are not always eliminated within the granuloma, but can become dormant, resulting in a latent infection. Another feature of the granulomas of human tuberculosis is the development of abnormal cell death, also called <u>necrosis</u>, in the center of <u>tubercles</u>. To the naked eye this has the texture of soft white cheese and was termed <u>caseous</u> <u>necrosis</u>.

If TB bacteria gain entry to the bloodstream from an area of damaged tissue they spread through the body and set up many foci of infection, all appearing as tiny white tubercles in the tissues. This severe form of TB disease is most common in infants and the elderly and is called <u>miliary tuberculosis</u>. Patients with this disseminated TB have a fatality rate near 100% if untreated. However, if treated early, the fatality rate is reduced to near 10%.

In many patients the infection waxes and wanes. Tissue destruction and necrosis are balanced by healing and <u>fibrosis</u>. Affected tissue is replaced by scarring and cavities filled with cheese-like white necrotic material. During active disease, some of these cavities are joined to the air passages <u>bronchi</u> and this material can be coughed up. It contains living bacteria and can therefore pass on infection. Treatment with appropriate <u>antibiotics</u> kills bacteria and allows healing to take place. Upon cure, affected areas are eventually replaced by scar tissue.

If untreated, infection with *Mycobacterium tuberculosis* can become <u>lobar pneumonia</u>.

TUBERCULOSIS DIAGNOSIS

The doctor will complete the following tests to diagnose tuberculosis. You may not be hospitalized for either the initial tests or the beginning of treatment.

- Chest X-ray: The most common diagnostic test that leads to the suspicion of infection is a <u>chest X-ray</u>.

  o In primary TB, an X-ray will show an abnormality in the mid and lower lung fields, and lymph nodes may be enlarged.

  o Reactivated TB bacteria usually <u>infiltrate</u> the upper lobes of the lungs.

- o Miliary tuberculosis exhibits diffuse nodules at different locations in the body.

- The Mantoux skin test also known as a tuberculin skin test (TST or PPD test): This test helps identify people infected with *M. tuberculosis* but who have no symptoms. A doctor must read the test.

  - o The doctor will inject 5 units of purified protein derivative (PPD) into your skin. If a raised bump of more than 5 mm (0.2 in) appears at the site 48 hours later, the test may be positive.

  - o This test can often indicate disease when there is none (false positive). Also, it can show no disease when you may in fact have TB (false negative).

- QuantiFERON-TB Gold test: This is a blood test that is an aid in the diagnosis of TB. This test can help detect active and latent tuberculosis. The body responds to the presence of the tuberculosis bacteria. By special techniques, the patient's blood is incubated with proteins from TB bacteria. If the bacteria are in the patient, the immune cells in the blood sample respond to these proteins with the production of a substance called interferon-gamma (IFN-gamma). This substance is detected by the test. If someone had a prior BCG vaccination (a vaccine against TB given in some countries but not the U.S.) and a positive skin test due to this, the QuantiFERON-TB Gold test will not detect any IFN-gamma.

- Sputum testing: Sputum testing for acid-fast bacilli is the only test that confirms a TB diagnosis. If sputum (the mucus you cough up) is available, or can be induced, a lab test may give a positive result in up to 30% of people with active disease.

  - o Sputum or other bodily secretions such as from your stomach or lung fluid can be cultured for growth of mycobacteria to confirm the diagnosis.

o It may take one to three weeks to detect growth in a culture, but eight to 12 weeks to be certain of the diagnosis.

TREATMENT

Treatment for TB uses antibiotics to kill the bacteria. Effective TB treatment is difficult, due to the unusual structure and chemical composition of the mycobacterial cell wall, which makes many antibiotics ineffective and hinders the entry of drugs. The two antibiotics most commonly used are rifampicin and isoniazid. However, instead of the short course of antibiotics typically used to cure other bacterial infections, TB requires much longer periods of treatment (around 6 to 24 months) to entirely eliminate mycobacteria from the body. Latent TB treatment usually uses a single antibiotic, while active TB disease is best treated with combinations of several antibiotics, to reduce the risk of the bacteria developing antibiotic resistance. People with latent infections are treated to prevent them from progressing to active TB disease later in life.

Drug-resistant tuberculosis is transmitted in the same way as regular TB. Primary resistance occurs in persons infected with a resistant strain of TB. A patient with fully susceptible TB develops secondary resistance (acquired resistance) during TB therapy because of inadequate treatment, not taking the prescribed regimen appropriately, or using low-quality medication. Drug-resistant TB is a public health issue in many developing countries, as treatment is longer and requires more expensive drugs. Multi-drug-resistant tuberculosis (MDR-TB) is defined as resistance to the two most effective first-line TB drugs: rifampicin and isoniazid. Extensively drug-resistant TB (XDR-TB) is also resistant to three or more of the six classes of second-line drugs.

The DOTS (Directly Observed Treatment Short-course) strategy of tuberculosis treatment recommended by WHO was based on clinical trials done in the 1970s by Tuberculosis Research Centre, Chennai, India. The country in which a person with TB lives can determine what treatment they receive. This is because multidrug-resistant tuberculosis is resistant to most first-line medications, the use of second-line anti tuberculosis medications is necessary to cure the patient. However, the price of these medications is high; thus poor people in the developing world have no or limited access to these treatments.

5.4 URINARY TRACT INFECTION

The urinary tract is the body's filtering system for removing liquid waste, or urine. It comprises the kidneys, ureters (tubes that carry urine from kidneys to bladder), bladder, and urethra (tube that carries urine from the bladder for excretion). A urinary tract infection (UTI) is caused by bacteria that enter the urinary tract.

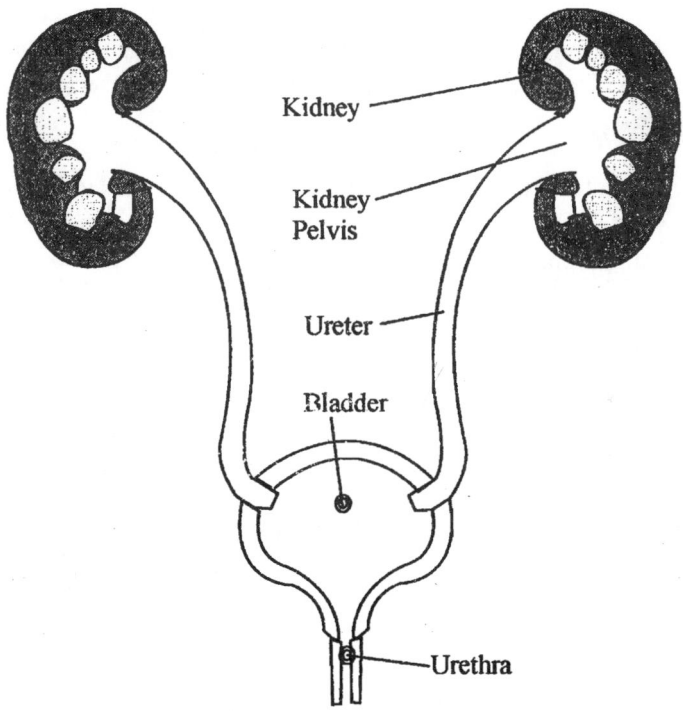

Fig.4. Urinary tract infection

Women are more likely than men to get UTIs because of their urinary tract's design. Men have a longer urethra, so it is more difficult for bacteria to enter the urinary tract. Nearly half of all women will have a urinary tract infection at some point in their lives. About 20 percent of these women will have repeat infections.

The urinary tract has two parts: the lower and upper tracts. Most infections occur in the lower urinary tract and can also be called bladder infections. Infections in the lower tract (involving the bladder and urethra) are more common because bacteria can easily enter this area.

Infections in the upper urinary tract (involving the kidneys and ureters) can also be called kidney infections and cause serious illness.

SYMPTOMS

Symptoms of a lower urinary tract infection or bladder infection may include:

- Frequent need to urinate
- Burning sensation while urinating
- Pressure in the lower abdomen
- Pain in the lower back
- Blood in urine

Symptoms of an upper urinary tract infection or a kidney infection may include:

- Fever
- Chills
- Nausea and/or vomiting
- Pain higher in the back (around the upper sides and waist)

In women, the symptoms of a urinary tract infection are similar to those caused by some vaginal infections.

CAUSES OF UTIS

In women, urinary tract infections usually are caused by bacteria that live on the skin near the rectum or vagina. These bacteria can travel through the urinary tract and cause infections in the bladder or other parts of the urinary tract. UTIs in men are rare and usually indicate an abnormal urinary tract or an enlarged prostate.

The most common causes of urinary tract infections are:

- *Sexual intercourse* - The back and forth motion of the penis during intercourse can push bacteria into the urethra. Bladder infections are more common in women who have had multiple sexual partners or have frequent intercourse.

- *Waiting too long to urinate* - The bladder is a muscle that gets bigger when it holds urine and shrinks to push it out. Waiting too long to urinate can cause the bladder muscles to stretch too much. Stretching weakens the muscle so not all the urine is pushed out, increasing the risk of a urinary tract infection.

Other causes include:

- Kidney stones that may physically block the free flow of urine

- Cystocele: relaxing of the bladder and vaginal area, which causes pools of urine to remain in the bladder

- Diverticular: infections that develop on the inside wall of the urethra, allowing urine to collect

- Urethral stenosis: a narrowing of the urethra, preventing an easy flow of urine out of the body - this can be present at birth or result from a number of conditions or activities

  Certain conditions may put you at risk for urinary tract infections, including

- Urinary tract infections in childhood

- Diabetes

- Pregnancy

TESTING FOR UTIS

Several methods may be used to tell whether you have a UTI.

- A urine sample may be used to evaluate the number of bacteria and white blood cells present. A high number of white blood cells in your urine may indicate an infection.

- A pelvic exam may be needed to rule out a vaginal or pelvic problem.

X-rays or ultrasounds may be used if infection returns often or does not respond to treatment.

TREATMENT

Urinary tract infections are treated with antibiotics. *It is very important to use all medication that your doctor prescribes, even if symptoms go away before finishing the medication.* Your doctor may recommend testing your urine after the treatment is finished to be sure the infection has completely cleared up.

If you have had several bladder infections, or even one kidney infection, your doctor may refer you to an urologist. An urologist is a doctor who specializes in treating problems of the urinary tract.

PREVENTION

You can help prevent urinary tract infections by practicing the following health habits:

- Understand the causes.

- Practice good personal hygiene. Always wipe from front to back.

- Drink plenty of fluids (at least three to four glasses of water each day) to help flush bacteria out of the urinary tract.

- Empty your bladder completely as soon as you feel the urge, or at least every three hours.

- Get plenty of vitamin C. It makes urine acidic and helps keep bacteria down. Vitamin C is found in orange juice, citrus fruits, and broccoli.

- Wear cotton underwear. Bacteria grow better in moist places. Cotton does not trap moisture.

- If you contract an infection, see your doctor and follow the prescribed treatment.

Several additional measures are helpful for women:

- During intercourse, try different positions that cause less friction between your urethra and your partner's penis.

- Change sanitary pads and tampons frequently during menstruation.

- After intercourse, urinate as soon as possible. This will help flush out any bacteria that may have gone into the urinary tract.

If you have any symptoms of a urinary tract infection, see a doctor as soon as possible. With proper treatment, the infection can be cleared up before it causes serious problems.

5.5 ENTERIC INFECTIONS

INTRODUCTION

The topic of enteric infections encompasses all infections of the intestinal tract. Certain infections have an anatomic preference, - causing disease of the esophagus, stomach, small intestine, or large intestine, while others can involve multiple anatomic areas of the intestinal tract or involve distant organs in addition to the intestines. While many systemic illnesses are caused by infectious agents that enter via the intestinal tract and disseminate, such as acute Hepatitis (Hepatitis A or Hepatitis B viruses) or Typhoid Fever (*Salmonella typhi*).

Susceptibility to certain infections is determined primarily by the status of the immune system of the individual, which can be greatly affected by immunosuppressive drugs (corticosteroids, cancer chemotherapy, 6-mercaptopurine, and tumor necrosis factor antagonists), organ transplantation, or HIV/AIDS. Water sources and sanitation, seasonality, environmental factors, as well as local outbreaks, determine risk of various infections geographically. Bacteria, yeast/fungi, viruses, and parasites (worms and amoeba-like protozoans) all cause enteric infections. The following table depicts the anatomic location and the various infectious agents that cause intestinal disease, provide an overview of clinical syndromes associated with the various infectious agents and give a general overview of standard first-line treatment for most infections.

Table 5. Important Definitions

Esophagitis	Inflammation of the lining of the esophagus
Gastritis	Inflammation of the lining of the stomach
Gastroenteritis	Inflammation of the lining of the stomach and small intestine resulting in acute diarrhea
Enterocolitis	Inflammation of both the lining of the small intestine and the large intestine (colon) resulting in severe diarrhea
Colitis	Inflammation of the lining of the large intestine (colon) resulting in severe diarrhea
Dysentery	Frequent, small-volume, severe bloody <u>diarrhea</u> often accompanied by <u>intestinal</u> <u>cramping</u>, fever, mailasie and <u>tenesmus</u> (painful straining and urgency to pass stool)
Proctitis	Inflammation of the anus and the distal rectum (anatomically the last part of the colon that connects the intestinal tract to the anus) resulting in pain and urgency and often bloody mucus drainage
Virus	A very small microbe that requires another organism to grow and reproduce
Bacteria	A small, free-living prokaryotic microbe
Protozoa	A free-living, relatively large, one-celled organism that is a complex eukaryote, the cell-type shared by higher organisms (e.g., amoeba)
Fungus	Eukaryotic organisms with a unique cell wall component (chitin) with various forms (yeast, mold, spores)

What are the causes of infectious esophagitis?

Infections of the esophagus are rarely seen in someone with a normal immune system. The most frequently diagnosed infection is candidal esophagitis, but herpes viruses and other viruses can occasionally infect the lining of the esophagus as well. Esophagitis is often seen in the setting of HIV/AIDS, hematologic malignancies (leukemia, lymphoma), cancer chemotherapy, long-term oral or inhaled corticosteroid or antibiotic use, and poorly controlled diabetes. Diagnosis of esophagitis without a known underlying condition should prompt further investigation of the immune status of the patient.

Candidal esophagitis is caused by members of the Candida species of yeast which includes Candida albicans, Candida glabrata, Candida parapsilosis, Candida tropicalis, Candida krusei and many others but Candida albicans accounts for the vast majority. Esophageal candidiasis can be accompanied by oropharyngeal candidiasis (termed "oral thrush") making the diagnosis of this infection much easier since it is easily visible to the health care provider. Oral thrush can be asymptomatic, but extensive candidal infection, as occurs with esophagitis, usually causes significant symptoms of pain and sharp discomfort, particularly with swallowing. It can occasionally cause nausea and vomiting as well. When present in the mouth, it appears as white plaques on the mucosal surfaces which can be sent for fungal wet prep (KOH) and culture for microbiologic confirmation. However, diagnosis of esophageal candidiasis without oral involvement generally requires upper endoscopy with culture and biopsy of plaque-like lesions. Pathology will show budding yeast with pseudohyphae invading mucosal surface cells. Treatment of candidiasis can vary depending on the immune status of the host, the extent of involvement of infection, and the species of Candida. *C. albicans* is almost always susceptible to first-line antifungal agents such as topical solution nystatin ("swish and swallow") which is used for prevention or mild disease or oral fluconazole for moderate-severe disease; resistance can emerge over time.

Several members of the **herpes family** can also cause disease of the esophagus. These viruses are often acquired early in life and persist in the body in latent form after initial exposure. When the immune system is suppressed, they can reactivate and can cause substantial morbidity and mortality in several parts of the body. Herpes simplex virus 1 and 2 (HSV-1 and HSV-2), Cytomegalovirus (CMV), and Varicella zoster virus (VZV) can all reactivate in the esophagus and cause extensive erosions and ulcerations. Diagnosis cannot be made based on simple visualization because they all cause an appearance of ulceration. These infections are often extremely painful and can lead to microscopic, although rarely substantial gastrointestinal bleeding. Diagnosis is made by upper endoscopy and biopsy which shows viral cytopathic effect, Cowdry intranuclear inclusions, and multinuclear giant cells (see images). Designated PCR testing (polymerase chain reaction) and viral culture will yield a specific viral diagnosis. HSV also causes gastrointestinal (GI) involvement of the lips, mouth, rectum, and peri-anal tissue (usually HSV-2 with genital/rectal and HSV-1 with oral and esophageal involvement). CMV can infect any part of the GI tract but is most commonly seen in the esophagus and large intestine and is a common cause of rectal bleeding and diarrhea, particularly in the setting of AIDS. Treatment of viral infections of the GI tract depends on the viral agent; an acyclovir-based regimen (acyclovir, valacyclovir or famciclovir) will treat HSV and VZV while CMV requires a ganciclovir-based therapy. It is not uncommon to have more than one pathogen identified at the time of diagnosis.

THE STOMACH

What are the causes of infectious gastritis?

The term gastritis refers to inflammation of the lining of the stomach, which can be caused by problems with acid regulation, drug effect (e.g., aspirin, non-steroidal anti-inflammatory agents), or infection. Because of the high level of acid in the stomach, few micro-organisms can survive and thrive in this environment.

Staphylococcus aureus or Bacillus cereus can thrive in the generally inhospitable environment of the stomach. These foodborne, toxin-mediated bacterial strains cause acute gastritis by releasing a toxin into the stomach, causing acute nausea and vomiting ("food poisoning"). They generally resolve rapidly without treatment-onset of symptoms is usually between 4-7 hours after the contaminated meal and resolution of symptoms is usually within 12 hours of onset of nausea and vomiting.

Helicobacter pylori is another bacterial pathogen that involves the stomach. This curved bacterium is able to tightly adhere to gastric epithelial cells and is protected from acid by hiding in the thick mucus layer. It has been associated with chronic infection of the stomach and duodenum leading to dyspepsia and peptic ulcer disease and rarely gastric malignancies.

THE INTESTINES

What is gastroenteritis and enterocolitis and what are the causes?

Gastroenteritis ("stomach flu") is an extremely most common illness, affecting approximately 11% of the United States population in a given year. The term gastroenteritis refers to inflammation of the lining of the intestinal tract of the stomach and small intestine, although the phrase is used indiscriminately, and many infections involve just the small intestine or the small and large intestine, termed "enterocolitis." While symptoms vary depending on the infectious agent, pathogens which primarily involve the small intestine, such as certain protozoa, viruses and cholera, typically cause watery diarrhea and mild abdominal cramps as well as nausea, vomiting, anorexia (loss of appetite) and dehydration. Most episodes of gastroenteritis are acquired by the fecal-oral route of transmission-this occurs when infected stool particles are transmitted via contamination of hands to another host who then ingests these particles and acquires infection. Many intermediary steps are usually required, including water that has come in contact with feces and is improperly treated before drinking, food that has been poorly handled, and poor sewage treatment.

Salmonella and *Yersinia* usually infect the distal ileum (the last part of the small intestine), but colonic (large intestine) involvement is common as well. Fever is often present and diarrhea may be watery or frankly bloody ("dysentery"). *Shigella, Campylobacter, E. histolytica* and CMV all cause colitis, with symptoms of lower abdominal pain, tenesmus (sensation of urgency to defecate), and fever. The stools are of smaller volume and contain blood and mucus. The majority of cases of acute infectious gastroenteritis are caused by viral pathogens, although bacteria and protozoans cause a substantial portion as well, particularly in the setting of foodborne outbreaks and in overseas traveler's diarrhea. In a review of approximately 30,000 bacterial stool cultures performed in the United States from 1990-1992, a bacterial cause was found in only 5.6% (1) of the samples, with the rest of the episodes attributed to viral or protozoal pathogens.

Because of the well-recognized clinical syndrome and the brief duration of illness, most episodes of acute gastroenteritis do not require precise diagnosis of the infectious agent; however determination of the etiology can be particularly important in the setting of an outbreak. Only a small fraction of stool samples submitted for culture or parasite detection yield a pathogen and patients are often asymptomatic by the time enteric pathogens are identified. Stool examination should be performed if severe or prolonged symptoms occur, fecal leukocytes in the stool (white blood cells which are a marker of colonic tissue invasion and an inflammatory process) are present, the patient is immunocompromised, or the patient has traveled and the gastroenteritis is not self-limited. Treatment for viral agents of disease is entirely supportive, with maintenance of hydration while bacterial and protozoal infections can be treated with targeted antibiotic therapy. The major infectious agents are described below (see table 4 for complete list):

Viruses

Noroviruses (e.g., Norwalk-like virus) account for foodborne outbreaks in diverse settings such as cruise ships, nursing homes, and hospitals, and are a common cause of overseas traveler's diarrhea. It is estimated that over one-third of outbreaks of non-bacterial gastroenteritis in the United States are caused by these viruses. The virus is highly infectious and requires only a small number of organisms to spread among people by the fecal-oral route. The incubation period is 24-48 hours and the average duration of symptoms is between 1-4 days, with characteristic explosive vomiting and diarrhea. The mechanism by which these viruses induce vomiting and diarrhea is not well understood.

Astroviruses have also been associated with outbreaks of gastroenteritis, predominantly in settings that involve children, such as in daycare centers and schools. It is more common in HIV-infected children or children with hematologic malignancies.

Rotavirus is the single most important cause of severe, dehydrating gastroenteritis in infants and children worldwide, and causes substantial morbidity and mortality in resource-poor settings where people do not have access to rapid rehydration through intravenous fluid resuscitation or oral rehydration therapy. Based on a recent meta-analysis, rotavirus is estimated to cause approximately 111 million episodes of gastroenteritis requiring only home care, 25 million clinic visits, 2 million hospitalizations, and 352,000–592,000 deaths (median, 440,000 deaths) in children <5 years of age. By age 5, nearly every child will have an episode of rotavirus gastroenteritis, 1 in 5 will visit a clinic, 1 in 65 will be hospitalized, and approximately 1 in 293 will die. Children in the poorest countries account for 82% of rotavirus deaths. Adolescents and adults are protected by development of protective antibodies when exposed in early childhood. A childhood vaccine against rotavirus (RotaTeq) was recently approved and implemented into routine pediatric care in the United States.

     Enteric adenovirus (serotypes 40 and 41) cause approximately 5-10% of pediatric gastroenteritis in the United States.

Bacteria

     Campylobacter jejuni accounts for approximately 2.3% of all episodes of gastroenteritis and close to 50% of all cases of bacterial gastroenteritis. It is most commonly acquired from undercooked contaminated poultry. Diarrhea is usually watery but can occasionally become hemorrhagic, and abdominal pain, cramping, and fever are often present. Unique to *C. jejuni* infection is its association with post-infectious reactive arthritis and Guillain-Barre syndrome, an ascending paralysis, felt to be caused by antibody cross-reactivity and auto-immunity.

     Salmonella enteritidis and *Salmonella typhimurium* are commonly associated with ingestion of poultry, eggs, and milk products as well as meats, contaminated fresh produce, and other food products. Additionally, several animals can transmit these bacteria, such as turtles. Like *C. jejuni*, *Salmonellosis* usually presents as watery diarrhea but can become hemorrhagic if colitis (inflammation of the large intestine) develops. Salmonella can infect all adults and children but certain factors put people at increased risk. These include lymphoproliferative disorders, young age, and altered intestinal flora due to surgery, inflammatory bowel disease, or recent antibiotic use. Rarely, these bacteria can enter the bloodstream and develop distant sites of infection in the bone (often associated with Sickle Cell Disease), the brain, or in the lining of the blood vessels (endovascular infection).

Shigella species are known as the classic cause of "dysentery," or bloody diarrhea. Shigella species cause infection with transmission of as few as 10 organisms and can spread by food or the fecal-oral route. Shigella produces a well-studied toxin, termed "shiga toxin" which can cause a systemic syndrome seen primarily in children called the "hemolytic uremic syndrome" that affects the blood cells, causing anemia and kidney damage.

Vibrio cholera, the etiologic agent of cholera infection, is an important cause of infectious diarrhea worldwide and leads to substantial mortality in locations where access to fluid resuscitation is not feasible. It is predominantly contracted via exposure to infected water. While cholera is not a problem currently in the United States, *Vibrio cholera* bacteria have been isolated in the Gulf of Mexico, and has caused epidemics in South America. *V. cholera* produces profuse watery diarrhea by release of a potent enterotoxin which inhibits salt absorption from the intestinal lining, leading to massive fluid secretion and loss into the gut lumen (3). The toxin produces virtually no inflammatory response. As with rotavirus, the cornerstones of management include estimation of the volume depletion and timely replacement of fluid and electrolyte deficits. This can be achieved by intravenous fluids or by the standard World Health Organization formula, available in packets, which includes sodium chloride, sodium bicarbonate, glucose, potassium chloride, and water. Antibiotic therapy with tetracycline may shorten the duration of illness and reduce shedding of the bacteria and further transmission. *Vibrio parahaemolyticu* is a cause of worldwide diarrheal disease and is found in coastal areas of the United States, where contaminated shellfish transmit the disease.

Escherichia coli species account for a number of gastrointestinal syndromes. Most *E. coli* species colonize the intestines and live as normal human gut flora. However, several toxins and unique virulence factors give different strains of *E. coli* the ability to cause human disease:

- *Enterotoxigenic E. coli:* causes watery diarrhea, and is the most common bacterial cause of traveler's diarrhea, mediated by release of a toxin similar to cholera toxin.

- *Enteropathogenic E. coli:* associated with infantile watery diarrhea.

- *Enterohemorrhagic E. coli:* causes a hemorrhagic colitis. The E. coli 0157:H7 serotype is associated with production of a toxin similar to the toxin of Shigella species, the "shiga-like" toxin, and is the most commonly identified cause of the hemolytic uremic syndrome (HUS) in the United States. Epidemics have been traced to contaminated beef but transmission through other food products, such as unpasteurized apple cider and raspberries (infected by contamination of animal feces), have also been reported. This has also been associated with petting zoos Antibiotics have not been shown to be helpful and potentially increase the risk of developing HUS, so should be avoided.

- *Enteroinvasive E. coli:* agent of travel diarrhea and dysentery.

- *Enteroaggregative E. coli:* agent that causes persistent diarrhea in children and people with AIDS.

Yersinia enterocolitica infection is most common in developed countries such as the United States, and is associated with water or foodborne outbreaks.

Clostridium perfringens is a cause of watery diarrhea. It is a foodborne toxin-mediated process caused by release of toxin from a large number of ingested bacteria. The spores of *C. perfringens* can germinate in many types of foods and can be associated with unhygienic canning procedures.

Listeria monocytogenes is a cause of abdominal pain, cramping, and diarrhea. It is seen primarily in immunocompromised individuals and is particularly harmful in the setting of pregnancy. The relative immunodeficiency in the third trimester puts women at 17-fold risk of disseminated infection and transmission to the fetus can result in stillbirth. It has been associated with outbreaks of deli meats and is commonly associated with unpasteurized dairy products. After ingestion, Listeria may cause isolated intestinal disease but also may disseminate to the bloodstream and distant organs such as the central nervous system, resulting in meningitis.

Protozoa

Cryptosporidium parvum is the most common parasitic cause of acute foodborne diarrhea in the United States. In the person with an intact immune system, Cryptosporidium causes severe dehydrating diarrhea that is self-limited. In people with AIDS or other immunocompromised hosts, it may become persistent and debilitating, particularly because there is no effective treatment other than correction of the host's immune system. Transmission occurs via spread from animals or humans or from contaminated food and water sources.

Giardia lamblia causes both epidemic and sporadic disease and is a common cause of water and foodborne diarrhea, particularly unfiltered water supplies, even if chlorinated. This is true even in fast flowing streams which can be contaminated by animal feces. As with Cryptosporidium, immunocompromised hosts can develop chronic recurrent giardiasis. The time course is prolonged, even in the normal host, with onset within 9-14 days and symptom resolution by 4-6 weeks. Many infections are asymptomatic but most have a mild watery diarrhea with or without cramping, flatulence, and malabsorption. Diagnosis is made by visualization of cysts in the stool or a stool antigen test. Treatment is with metronidazole 250 mg three times daily for 10 days but there is an 8-20% failure rate.

Entamoeba histolytica is a worldwide cause of infectious enterocolitis and is more prevalent in areas with poor sanitary conditions, infecting up to 10% of the world's population. In the United States, it is more commonly seen as an infectious agent in migrant workers from Central America, overseas travelers, and in men who have sex with men. Symptoms range from asymptomatic carrier state to mild diarrhea to severe dysentery. Symptoms are slow to develop, ranging from 1-3 weeks, and can persist for several weeks to months. In severe cases, toxic megacolon may develop with fulminant colitis which may lead to perforation. A rare complication is the development of amoebomas (tumor-like masses in the lining of the intestinal tract), which may cause intestinal obstruction and can be palpated on physical examination. Liver abscess is a common complication, often seen in people who never had intestinal symptoms. The abscess is usually found as a solitary mass in the right lobe of the liver. Ultrasound or computer tomographic imaging will reveal a hepatic abscess without specific characteristics but aspiration of contents will reveal trophozoites consistent with Entamoeba infection. Diagnosis of intestinal amoebiasis can be made by simple stool examination for characteristic cysts or by blood test for entamoeba antibody. In the setting of colitis, colonoscopy reveals involvement of the cecum (the last part of the small intestine which connects to the large intestine) and colon with characteristic "flask" ulcers with a wider base beneath the superficial epithelium. Biopsy reveals classic trophozoites, necrotic debris and eosinophil cells.

Cyclospora cayetanensis has been associated with outbreaks of contaminated raspberries and basil. It causes a small intestine watery diarrhea. Like giardiasis, infection with Cyclospora may cause several weeks of symptoms, which can include fatigue and malaise in addition to diarrhea. Cyclospora can develop a chronic unrelenting infection in the setting of AIDS and other conditions that inhibit the immune system. Cyclospora is easily treated with trimethoprim-sulfamethoxazole for 7-10 days but relapse may occur. Isospora and Microsporidia are two other infectious parasites that cause a clinical syndrome similar to Cryptosporidia and Cyclospora, and are also more commonly seen in the setting of immunosuppression and AIDS. Isospora is also treated with trimethoprim-sulfamethoxazole and Microsporidia with albendazole for a prolonged course (up to 3 months). For all of these infections, diagnosis can be made based on examination of stool cysts which each have a characteristic appearance and for staining with an acid-fast stain.

THE ANUS AND RECTUM

What infections cause proctitis?

Proctitis is infection and inflammation of the rectum and anus. Sexually transmitted infections such as **herpes** (Herpes simplex virus), **syphilis** (*Treponema pallidum*), **genital warts** (condyloma acuminata, caused by Human papilloma virus) **gonorrhea** (*Neisseria gonorrhea*) and **chlamydia** (*Chlamydia trachomatis*) are introduced into the rectum during anal intercourse and cause rectal and anal disease that may be asymptomatic or may cause symptoms of purulent discharge, pain, itching, and rectal bleeding. Diagnosis, in certain circumstances, can be made by culture of adherent mucus. Treatment is the same as for genital involvement.

Lymphogranularum venereum (LGV) (caused by a specific serovar of *Chlamydia trachomatis*) causes persistent infection with fever and enlargement of local lymph nodes, which may suppurate and form tracts into other tissues if untreated. Anal ulcerations and strictures may be mistaken for Crohn's disease. LGV is diagnosed by specific antibody detection and requires 3 weeks of treatment with doxycycline or tetracycline.

What other important diseases of the intestinal tract are there?

Many other infections affect the intestinal tract. Four important infectious agents that do not fit well into other classifications include *Mycobacterium tuberculosis, Mycobacterium avium intracellulare, Histoplasma capsulatum and Clostridium difficile.*

Mycobacterium tuberculosis (or rarely *Mycobacterium bovis*) infects the gastrointestinal tract after ingested organisms penetrate normal mucosa. This is an uncommon manifestation of tuberculosis which is predominantly a pulmonary disease, although tuberculosis can affect the lymph nodes, brain, kidneys, uterus, and many other organs. Gastrointestinal tuberculosis can cause fever, gastrointestinal bleeding, abdominal pain, and weight loss and can result in ulceration, stricture, mass lesions (tubercles), and fistula formation. Thickening of the bowel and lymphadenopathy are often present. The cecum and terminal ileum are most commonly infected, but any part of the intestinal tract can be involved. Disease is often segmental and mimics Crohn's disease. Histologically, necrotizing granulomas with acid-fast bacilli confirm the diagnosis.

Mycobacterium Avium Complex (MAC) infection is a common manifestation of end-stage AIDS. MAC involves the gastrointestinal tract as part of a systemic infection of the blood and lymph nodes. It rarely causes serious infection in immunocompetent individuals. MAC infection causes watery diarrhea, abdominal cramping, fever, and weight loss. Diagnosis is made by culture of blood or stool and treatment requires a prolonged course of a macrolide-based regimen that often requires 2 or 3 antibiotics followed by preventive treatment with azithromycin until the immune system can be restored by the administration of HIV medications.

Histoplasma capsulatum is a fungus found in the soil of certain geographic locations, such as the central river valleys in the United States and parts of Central and South America. Infection follows inhalation of spores and lung disease is the most common site of infection. However, in the setting of immunosuppression, the fungus can spread throughout the body including the brain and has a predilection for the gastrointestinal tract where it can cause ulcerations and rectocolitis. The mouth is also a common site of disease, with ulcerations and mass-like lesions that can be mistaken for oral cancer. Diagnosis is made based on culture of blood, bone marrow, or lymph node, by biopsy showing classic intracellular organisms and non-caseating granulomas, or by antigen (urine and blood) or antibody test. Therapy for disseminated histoplasmosis depends on whether or not the brain and meninges are involved. It requires a prolonged course of intravenous amphotericin, followed by oral itraconazole indefinitely, until the immune system of the individual can be restored by cancer or HIV treatment.

Clostridium difficile is a hardy, spore-forming bacterium that emerges as an important pathogen following administration of antibiotics. Clindamycin and ampicillin were most strongly indicted in early studies but virtually every antibiotic has been associated with *C. difficile* colitis. In recent years, the fluoroquinolone class of antibiotics (levofloxacin, ciprofloxacin, moxifloxacin) has become an important cause. *C. difficile* causes disease by release of its toxins, which are directly toxic to the lining of the intestinal tract, causing fluid loss and severe inflammation. Severe disease results in pseudo membranous colitis in which the lesions appear whitish-yellow with plaques and nodules consisting of necrotic cells visualized by colonoscopy. Antibiotics presumably induce *C. difficile* colitis by suppressing normal gut flora and allowing *C. difficile* to grow, colonize, and produce toxin. Although people in the community may be colonized, acquisition in the hospital setting is much more common. The diagnosis can be delayed because of the confusion with the mild form of diarrhea that is commonly induced by use of antibiotics. Culture of the stool for *C. difficile* is not useful due to the presence of many non-toxin producing strains that may inhabit the colon. Therefore, diagnosis is made by various tests looking directly for the toxin (agglutination ELISA tests, stool cytotoxin assay). Treatment includes discontinuation of the offending antibiotic (if possible) and a 10-14-day course of oral metronidazole or vancomycin. Relapse is common.

What helminthes (worms) infect the intestinal tract and what symptoms do they cause?

Several environmental helminthes can cause significant gastrointestinal disease as part of their life cycle. Symptoms and severity depend on the particular organisms and the stage of disease that involves the intestinal tract. All of these infestations occur by exposure through skin or by ingestion of contaminated food and water, thus the importance of wearing shoes when walking in moist soil, avoidance of swimming in ponds and lakes exposed to sewage, and avoidance of ingestion of fruit, vegetables, or local water in areas with poor sanitary standards. Some of the more common helminthes that cause human disease involving the gut are discussed below:

Anisakiasis is caused by ingestion of raw or improperly cooked seafood containing larvae of *Anisakidae*. Many seafood are infected and humans are accidental hosts. Ingestion can result in trivial infestation of the esophagus and throat, or in mucosal invasion of the stomach and intestine. Symptoms of invasive disease are usually rapid in onset and include abdominal pain, nausea, vomiting, and hives. Endoscopy is required for both diagnosis and treatment (removal of the larvae). Chronic infestation can cause eosinophilic granulomas. No specific medication is known to be effective in treatment of anisakiasis.

Strongyloidiasis is caused by the ubiquitous nematode (round worm). *Strongyloides stercoralis* which is found around the world, primarily in temperate climates, including the warmer parts of the United States. Strongyloides inhabits moist soil which can penetrate skin or be ingested. The larvae ultimately penetrate the small intestinal mucosa where they mature into adult worms that ultimately produce eggs that pass into the feces. A cycle of auto-infection via the skin of the anal region creates the potential for decades of infection; in immunocompromised hosts, a syndrome of "hyperinfection" can develop which can be fatal. Uncomplicated strongyloidiasis usually causes no symptoms; occasionally abdominal cramping, watery diarrhea, and malabsorption may develop. The changes of ulceration, stenosis, and mucosal fold thickening may be mistaken for Crohn's Disease. Diagnosis can be made upon finding larvae in the stool or tissues or by antibody blood test. Treatment depends on the clinical syndrome and several parasitic antibiotics may be effective.

Ascaris lumbricoides, a large roundworm found throughout the world, infects more than one billion people. Humans are infected when fertilized eggs are ingested by infected water or food sources. Mature eggs hatch in the duodenum (first part of small intestine), then penetrate the lymphatic system, travel to the lungs, up the bronchial tree and are then swallowed back into the intestinal tract. There, the adults mature and lay huge numbers of eggs. Most patients are asymptomatic, although lung symptoms can occur during the pulmonary phase, and heavy infestation of the gut can cause intestinal obstruction or migrate into the pancreas and liver. Diagnosis can be made on endoscopy, bronchoscopy (by visualization of larvae in the lungs), or by passing of the adult worms in the stool. Treatment is with albendazole.

Whipworm, or *Trichuris trichiura,* are easily identified in stool specimens. Infection occurs by ingestion of embryonated eggs in contaminated food or water which directly hatch in the small intestine. Symptoms are usually absent and treatment is also with albendazole or mebendazole.

Hookworm is caused by two worms, *Necator americanus* and *Ancylostoma duodenale* which live in mammals such as cats and dogs. Both larvae can penetrate skin with migration via the venous system to the lungs and back to the intestinal system, as seen in ascariasis above. Abdominal pain and anemia may ensue but the majority of people are asymptomatic. Treatment is with albendazole.

Enterobius vermicularis, or **pinworm**, is a small, threadlike worm that enjoys a worldwide distribution, including cosmopolitan regions. It is most often seen in children. Adult worms live primarily in the cecum (last part of the small intestine) but migrate at night to the perianal region, where they deposit eggs, which cause intense itching. Eggs are immediately infectious so household spread is common. Diagnosis is made by the "scotch tape" test which demonstrates microscopic eggs from the perianal region. Treatment is with albendazole or mebendazole.

What intestinal infections are associated with HIV/AIDS?

Chronic diarrhea is a common clinical feature of patients with HIV/AIDS. Often, HIV medications account for intestinal symptoms of diarrhea, nausea, and cramping, however the cell-mediated immunodeficiency caused by advanced HIV infection/AIDS predisposes patients to several infectious pathogens. Several studies from the pre-HIV treatment era found that Cryptosporidia and cytomegalovirus were the most frequently encountered cause of infectious diarrhea, followed by Salmonella, Mycobacterium avium complex (MAC), and Entamoeba histolytica, respectively. Giardiasis, Herpes simplex esophagitis and proctitis, Campylobacter, Candidiasis, Histoplasmosis, Cyclospora, Isospora, and Microspora also cause substantial infection in those with HIV/AIDS (8-10). Kaposi's sarcoma, a vascular tumor seen much more commonly in the setting of HIV/AIDS, is associated with the Kaposi's sarcoma virus (KSV, also called Human Herpes virus 8 HHV-8) can involve any part of the intestinal tract as well (see image). *Mycobacterium tuberculosis* causes active and disseminated infection in the setting of HIV/AIDS and can involve the intestinal tract as well. In large cohort studies, over one third of patients were found to be simultaneously infected with more than one infectious agent. The rate of opportunistic infections, including the many causes of enteric infections listed above, are much less commonly seen in people who have access to HIV medications and whose immune systems are better preserved.

REVIEW QUESTIONS

ESSAY QUESTIONS

1. a.Classify oral anti-diabetic drugs with examples.
   b.Describe the pharmacological action of Glibenclamide and Phenformin.
2. Describe the terms Hyperthyroidism and Hypothyroidism and add a brief note on their treatment.
3. Name the drugs used in the treatment of UTIs and describe the pharmacological actions of any one of them.
4. Describe the chemotherapy of Urinary tract Infection and their rationale use.
5. Write short notes on Diabetes mellitus.
6. Enumerate Endocrine disorders and write on one of their treatment.

SHORT ANSWER QUESTIONS

7. Write about the diagnosis , symptoms and treatment of Tuberculosis.
8. Name the drugs used in the treatment of UTIs.
9. Describe the pharmacological action of Voglibose.
10. What are various Endocrine disorders?
11. Write about the chemotherapy of Gonorrhoea.
12. Write the treatment of any one endocrine disorder.

Chapter 6

HEMATOPOIETIC DISORDERS

6.1 ANEMIA

What is anemia?

Anemia is a blood disorder that is defined as:

- A level of red blood cells (RBCs) that is below the normal range, or

- A level of hemoglobin, the oxygen-carrying protein in RBCs, that is below normal.

There are several forms of anemia including:

- Iron deficiency anemia

- Hemolytic anemia (destruction of RBCs)

- Vitamin B-12 deficiency anemia

- Folic acid deficiency anemia

- Anemias caused by inherited abnormalities of RBCs (for example, sickle cell anemia and thalassemia)

- Anemia caused by chronic (ongoing) disease.

How do the different forms of anemia occur?

Iron deficiency anemia:

This most common form of anemia is caused by blood loss. Women most often develop iron deficiency anemia from the loss of blood during their menstrual periods and from repeated pregnancies. This type of anemia may also develop as a result of internal bleeding in the stomach (as with ulcers) or in the intestine (as with colon cancer). Iron deficiency anemia can also be caused by a lack of iron in the diet. Pregnant women may have this form of anemia because the growing fetus draws upon the mother's iron for the development of red blood cells and other tissues.

Hemolytic anemia:

This kind of anemia occurs when red blood cells are destroyed or damaged by infection, drugs, or inherited conditions.

Vitamin B-12 (cobalamin) deficiency anemia:

This type of anemia results from an inability of the stomach or intestines to absorb vitamin B-12. For example, an immune system disorder called pernicious anemia prevents normal absorption of the vitamin by the intestinal tract. Gastrointestinal illness, certain medications, and some inherited disorders may also cause vitamin B-12 deficiency. Some vegetarians may not get enough vitamin B-12 from the foods they eat. Besides causing anemia, a lack of vitamin B-12 affects the nervous system and may first cause symptoms of numbness, tingling, balance problems, depression, or memory difficulties.

Folic acid deficiency anemia:

Anemia due to a lack of folic acid in the diet is similar to B-12 deficiency anemia, but there is no damage to specific nerves. However, it can cause depression. This anemia is common in:

- Alcoholics, who often suffer from malnutrition

- Pregnant women

- People with intestinal malabsorption problems

- People using some daily medications, such as phenytoin, sulfasalazine, and possibly oral contraceptives.

Anemia caused by inherited abnormalities of RBCs:

Among several types of anemia caused by inherited abnormalities of RBCs, the most common are sickle cell anemia and thalassemia. Sickle cell anemia is an inherited disease predominantly of the black race. This anemia is characterized by abnormal hemoglobin structure and sickle-shaped RBCs. The abnormal sickle-shaped RBCs are damaged or destroyed as they pass through the circulatory system. The anemia usually has many noticeable effects on the person with this disease. It can cause a condition called sickle cell crisis. The crisis may occur under certain conditions such as altitude or pressure changes, low oxygen, or some illnesses. In sickle cell crisis the RBCs become even more deformed and block tiny blood vessels, causing acute, prolonged pain and other complications. Thalassemias are a group of inherited anemias caused by abnormal hemoglobin. The abnormal hemoglobin may cause abnormal red blood cells as well as low hemoglobin levels. Thalassemias most commonly affect people of Mediterranean descent, but some types also affect peoples of Africa, Asia, India, and the South Pacific. Most forms of thalassemia are mild, but some forms cause disease in children and may result in death before adulthood. People who have thalassemia should not take iron medication.

Anemia caused by disease:

Anemia caused by ongoing (chronic) disease is common in people who have:

- Cancer
- Leukemia
- Inflammatory diseases, such as rheumatoid arthritis
- Ongoing infections
- Kidney disease

What are the symptoms?

Mild anemia usually does not produce symptoms. More severe anemia is associated with:

- Weakness
- Fatigue
- Pale skin, gums, skin creases, and nailbeds.

Other symptoms of worsening anemia include:

- Lightheadedness
- Rapid heartbeat
- Shortness of breath, fainting
- Chest pain
- Heart failure.

Jaundice (yellow skin and eyes) may be a symptom of hemolytic anemia.

How is it treated?

The treatment depends on the type of anemia you have. Your doctor will check your blood count periodically to monitor the effect of your treatment.

Iron deficiency anemia:

To treat iron deficiency anemia (if there is no underlying disease causing blood loss), the doctor will simply prescribe iron supplements and/or a diet of foods rich in iron. Iron tablets may have side effects such as abdominal cramping; nausea; constipation; and dark, hard stools. To minimize side effects, your doctor will start you on a low dose of iron and slowly increase your dose to the necessary amount. He or she may suggest that you take vitamin C with the iron pills to help your body absorb the iron. Taking the iron at mealtimes can help prevent stomach and intestinal upset. Do not take antacids and do not eat or drink any dairy products at the same time you take the iron pills. Antacids and dairy products prevent the body from absorbing iron. Only rarely are iron injections necessary.

Vitamin B-12 deficiency anemia:

If you have this form of anemia because your stomach does not absorb vitamin B-12 well, the usual treatment is an injection of vitamin B-12 once a month. Sometimes an oral form (tablet) is used, but it must be taken in very high doses with a doctor's recommendation.

Folic acid deficiency anemia:

The treatment for folic acid deficiency anemia is daily oral folate tablets. This anemia is similar to vitamin B-12 deficiency anemia. Your doctor will not begin treatment with folate until he or she makes sure that your anemia is not caused by vitamin B-12 deficiency.

Anemia caused by inherited abnormalities of RBCs:

Sickle cell anemia usually requires frequent complex treatments. Sickle cell crisis requires intravenous fluids, rest, pain relief, and sometimes a blood transfusion. The treatment for thalassemias depends on such factors as the severity of the anemia, your age, and the risk of blood transfusions. When blood transfusions are needed for acute anemia, there is a small risk of acquiring blood-borne diseases such as hepatitis or AIDS, even though donated blood is carefully screened. Therefore, your doctor will recommend a transfusion only when it is clearly the best treatment for you. People who have thalassemia must not take iron medication.

Anemia caused by chronic disease:

Fortunately, the effects of this type of anemia usually tend to be mild. For certain conditions, such as chronic kidney disease, your doctor may prescribe regular injections of erythropoietin to stimulate your body's production of red blood cells.

How do I prevent anemia?

There are steps you can take to help prevent some types of anemia.

(a)   Eat foods high in iron:

- Cereal/breads with iron in it (100% iron-fortified is best. Check food label.)
- Liver
- Lentils and beans
- Oysters
- Tofu

- Green, leafy vegetables such as spinach

- Red meat (lean only)

- Fish

- Dried fruits such as apricots, prunes, and raisins

(b) Eat and drink foods that help your body absorb iron, like orange juice, strawberries, broccoli, or other fruits and vegetables with vitamin C.

(c) Don't drink coffee or tea with meals. These drinks make it harder for your body to absorb iron.

(d) Calcium can hurt your absorption of iron. If you have a hard time getting enough iron, talk to your doctor about the best way to also get enough calcium.

(e) Make sure you consume enough folic acid and vitamin B12.

(f) Make balanced food choices. Most people who make healthy, balanced food choices get the iron and vitamins their bodies need from the foods they eat. Food fads and dieting can lead to anemia.

(g) Talk to your doctor about taking iron pills (supplements). Do NOT take these pills without talking to your doctor first. These pills come in two forms: ferrous and ferric. The ferrous form is better absorbed by your body. But taking iron pills can cause side effects, like nausea, vomiting, constipation, and diarrhea. Reduce these side effects by taking these steps:

- Start with half of the recommended dose. Gradually increase to the full dose.

- Take the pill in divided doses. For example, if you are prescribed two pills daily, take one in morning with breakfast and the other after dinner.

- Take the pill with food.

- If one type of iron pill is causing problems, ask your doctor for another brand.

It is important to keep iron pills tightly capped and away from children's reach. In children, death has occurred from ingesting 200 mg of iron.

(h) If you are a non-pregnant woman of childbearing age, get tested for anemia every five to 10 years. This can be done during a regular health exam. Testing should start in adoles-cence.

(i) If you are a non-pregnant woman of childbearing age with these risk factors for iron deficiency, get tested every year:

- Heavy periods

- Low iron intake

- Have been diagnosed with anemia in the past

(j) Follow your doctor's orders for treating the underlying cause of your anemia. This will prevent the ane-mia from coming back or becoming serious.

PART B JOINT AND CONNECTIVE TISSUE DISORDERS

6.2 RHEUMATIC DISEASES

Rheumatic diseases can be defined as "disorders of connective tissue, especially the joints and related structures, characterized by inflammation, degeneration, or metabolic derangement.

Rheumatic diseases involve the joints, muscles, bones, tendons and other structures of the locomotor system. They can be inflammatory, degenerative or metabolic and comprise a range of disorders such as the different forms of arthritis, osteoporosis or connective tissue diseases.

SYMPTOMS

Different rheumatic diseases have different symptoms. In general, they are characterized by:

- Inflammation (signs of which are redness and/or heat, swelling, and pain)

- Loss of function of one or more connecting or supporting structures of the body

Common symptoms are pain, swelling, and stiffness. They especially affect joints, tendons, ligaments, bones, and muscles. Some rheumatic diseases can also involve internal organs.

DEVELOPING RHEUMATIC DISEASES - RISK FACTORS

- The causes of many of the rheumatic diseases are not sufficiently known and scientists are currently studying risk factors that increase the likelihood of developing a rheumatic disease.

- Some of these factors have been identified and many rheumatic diseases are believed to be affected by lifestyle factors such as:

  - Obesity

  - Smoking

  - Lack of physical activity

- In osteoarthritis, inherited cartilage weakness or excessive stress on the joint from repeated injury may play a role.

- In systemic lupus erythematosus (SLE), rheumatoid arthritis, and scleroderma, the combination of genetic factors that determine susceptibility and environmental triggers are believed to be important. Family history also plays a role in some diseases such as gout and ankylosing spondylitis.

- Gender is another factor in some rheumatic diseases. SLE, rheumatoid arthritis, scleroderma, and fibromyalgia are more common among women. This indicates that hormones or other male-female differences may play a role in the development of these conditions.

- Additionally, arthritis and other rheumatic diseases are often mistakenly associated with old age, because osteoarthritis (the most common form of arthritis) occurs more often amongst the elderly. However, arthritis and other rheumatic diseases affect people of all ages. Even babies and children can develop some forms of rheumatic disease.

Diagnosis

- Diagnosing rheumatic diseases can be difficult because some symptoms and signs are common to many different diseases.

- Whilst some rheumatic diseases can be identified by a physician based on symptoms and patient history, a diagnosis may often need to be confirmed in a hospital setting using sophisticated biochemical marker tests and imaging techniques.

- For some rheumatic diseases, such as inflammatory arthritis, it has become clear that early treatment helps to prevent or slow disease progression.

- Therefore early access to diagnostic assessments and disease-modifying therapies is a key part of the treatment strategy.

Treatment

- Most rheumatic diseases cannot be 'cured', however they can be managed in many cases so that symptoms do not impact on the patient's daily life. Both pharmacological and non-pharmacological therapies are important parts of a complete management programme for patients with rheumatic diseases.

- Non-pharmacological treatment includes rest and relaxation, exercise, dietary modifications, medication, and instruction about the proper use of joints and ways to conserve energy. Other treatments include the use of pain relief methods and assistive devices, such as splints or braces.

- In severe cases, surgery may be necessary. The doctor and the patient work together to develop a treatment plan that helps the patient maintain or improve his or her quality of life. Treatment plans usually combine several types of treatment and vary depending on the rheumatic condition and the patient.

- In Europe, several centres of excellence have been created which have made remarkable progress in studying rheumatic diseases over the last few years. European research has allowed the development of biological therapies in this field

6.3 HYPERURICEMIA

Hyperuricemia (British English: *hyperuricaemia*) is a level of uric acid in the blood that is abnormally high. In humans, the upper end of the normal range is 360 µmol/L (6 mg/dL) for women and 400 µmol/L (6.8 mg/dL) for men.

Causes

Many factors contribute to hyperuricemia, including: genetics, insulin resistance, hypertension, renal insufficiency, obesity, diet, use of diuretics, and consumption of alcoholic beverages. Of these, alcohol consumption is the most important.

Causes of hyperuricemia can be classified into three functional types: increased production of uric acid, decreased excretion of uric acid, and mixed type. Causes of increased production include high levels of purine in the diet and increased purine metabolism. Causes of decreased excretion include kidney disease, certain drugs, and competition for excretion between uric acid and other molecules. Mixed causes include high levels of alcohol and/or fructose in the diet, and starvation.

Increased production

A purine-rich diet is a common but minor cause of hyperuricemia. Diet alone generally is not sufficient to cause hyperuricemia. Purine content of foods varies. Foods high in the purines adenine and hypoxanthine may be more potent in exacerbating hyperuricemia.

Hyperuricemia of this type is a common complication of solid organ transplant. Apart from normal variation (with a genetic component), tumor lysis syndrome produces extreme levels of uric acid, mainly leading to renal failure. The Lesch-Nyhan syndrome is also associated with extremely high levels of uric acid.

Decreased excretion

The principal drugs that contribute to hyperuricemia by decreased excretion are the primary antiuricosurics. Other drugs and agents include diuretics, salicylates, pyrazinamide, ethambutol, nicotinic acid, ciclosporin, 2-ethylamino-1,3,4-thiadiazole, and cytotoxic agents.

The gene SLC2A9 encodes a protein that helps to transport uric acid in the kidney. Several single nucleotide polymorphisms of this gene are known to have a significant correlation with blood uric acid.

A ketogenic diet impairs the ability of the kidney to excrete uric acid, due to competition for transport between uric acid and ketones.

Elevated blood lead is significantly correlated with both impaired kidney function and hyperuricemia. In a study of over 2500 people resident in Taiwan, a blood lead level exceeding 7.5 µg/dL had odds ratios of 1.92 (95% CI: 1.18-3.10) for renal dysfunction and 2.72 (95% CI: 1.64-4.52) for hyperuricemia.

Mixed

Causes of hyperuricemia that are of "mixed" ("double whammy") type have a dual action, both increasing production and decreasing excretion of uric acid.

High intake of alcohol (ethanol), a significant cause of hyperuricemia, has a dual action that is compounded by multiple mechanisms. Ethanol increases production of uric acid by increasing production of lactic acid, hence lactic acidosis. Ethanol also increases the plasma concentrations of hypoxanthine and xanthine via the acceleration of adenine nucleotide degradation, and is a possible weak inhibitor of xanthine dehydrogenase. As a byproduct of its fermentation process, beer additionally contributes purines. Ethanol decreases excretion of uric acid by promoting dehydration and (rarely) clinical ketoacidosis.

High dietary intake of fructose contributes significantly to hyperuricemia. In a large study in the United States, consumption of four or more sugar-sweetened soft drinks per day gave an odds ratio of 1.82 for hyperuricemia. Increased production of uric acid is the result of interference, by a product of fructose metabolism, in purine metabolism. This interference has a dual action, both increasing the conversion of ATP to inosine and hence uric acid and increasing the synthesis of purine. Fructose also inhibits the excretion of uric acid, apparently by competing with uric acid for access to the transport protein SLC2A9. The effect of fructose in reducing excretion of uric acid is increased in people with a hereditary (genetic) predisposition toward hyperuricemia and/or gout.

Starvation causes the body to metabolize its own (purine-rich) tissues for energy. Thus, like a high purine diet, starvation increases the amount of purine converted to uric acid. A very low calorie diet without carbohydrate can induce extreme hyperuricemia; including some carbohydrate (and reducing the protein) reduces the level of hyperuricemia. Starvation also impairs the ability of the kidney to excrete uric acid, due to competition for transport between uric acid and ketones.

Treatment

Precipitation of uric acid crystals, and conversely their dissolution, is known to be dependent on the concentration of uric acid in solution, pH, sodium concentration, and temperature. Established treatments address these parameters.

Concentration

Following Le Chatelier's principle, lowering the blood concentration of uric acid may permit any existing crystals of uric acid to be gradually dissolved into the blood, from whence the dissolved uric acid can be excreted. Maintaining a lower blood concentration of uric acid similarly should reduce the formation of new crystals. If the person has chronic gout or known tophi, then large quantities of uric acid crystals may have accumulated in joints and other tissues, and aggressive and/or long duration use of medications may be needed.

Medications most often used to treat hyperuricemia are of two kinds: xanthine oxidase inhibitors and uricosurics. Xanthine oxidase inhibitors decrease the production of uric acid, by interfering with xanthine oxidase. Uricosurics increase the excretion of uric acid, by reducing the reabsorption of uric acid once the kidneys have filtered it out of the blood. Some of these medications are used as indicated; others are used off-label. Several other kinds of medications have potential for use in treating hyperuricemia. In people receiving hemodialysis, sevelamer can significantly reduce serum uric acid, apparently by adsorbing urate in the gut. In women, use of combined oral contraceptive pills is significantly associated with lower serum uric acid.

Non-medication treatments for hyperuricemia include a low purine diet and a variety of dietary supplements. These treatments are regarded by many physicians as having little or no efficacy. Treatment with lithium salts has been used as lithium improves uric acid solubility.

pH

Serum pH is neither safely nor easily altered. Therapies that alter pH principally alter the pH of urine, to discourage a possible complication of uricosuric therapy: formation of uric acid kidney stones due to increased uric acid in the urine. Dietary supplements that can be used to make the urine more alkaline include sodium bicarbonate, potassium citrate, magnesium citrate, and Shohl's Solution. Medications that have a similar effect include acetazolamide.

Temperature

Low temperature is a commonly reported trigger of acute gout: an example would be a day spent standing in cold water, followed by an attack of gout the next morning. This is believed to be due to temperature-dependent precipitation of uric acid crystals in tissues at below normal temperature. Thus, one aim of prevention is to keep the hands and feet warm, and soaking in hot water may be therapeutic.

6.4 GOUT

Gout (also known as **podagra** when it involves the big toe) is a medical condition usually characterized by recurrent attacks of acute inflammatory arthritis-a red, tender, hot, swollen joint. The metatarsal-phalangeal joint at the base of the big toe is the most commonly affected (~50% of cases). However, it may also present as tophi, kidney stones, or urate nephropathy. It is caused by elevated levels of uric acid in the blood which crystallize and are deposited in joints, tendons, and surrounding tissues.

Diagnosis is confirmed clinically by the visualization of the characteristic crystals in joint fluid. Treatment with nonsteroidal anti-inflammatory drugs (NSAIDs), steroids, or colchicine improves symptoms. Once the acute attack has subsided, levels of uric acid are usually lowered via lifestyle changes, and in those with frequent attacks allopurinol or probenicid provide long-term prevention.

Signs and Symptoms

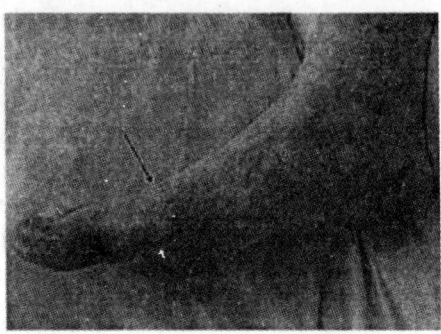

Fig.1. Gout presenting in the metatarsal-phalangeal joint of the big toe.

Gout can present in a number of ways, although the most usual is a recurrent attack of acute inflammatory arthritis (a red, tender, hot, swollen joint). The metatarsal-phalangeal joint at the base of the big toe is affected most often, accounting for half of cases. Other joints, such as the heels, knees, wrists and fingers, may also be affected. Joint pain usually begins over 2-4 hours and during the night. The reason for onset at night is due to the lower body temperature then. Other symptoms that may occur along with the joint pain include fatigue and a high fever.

Long-standing elevated uric acid levels (hyperuricemia) may result in other symptomatology, including hard, painless deposits of uric acid crystals known as tophi. Extensive tophi may lead to chronic arthritis due to bone erosion. Elevated levels of uric acid may also lead to crystals precipitating in the kidneys, resulting in stone formation and subsequent urate nephropathy.

Causes

Hyperuricemia is the underlying cause of gout. This can occur for a number of reasons, including diet, genetic predisposition, or under excretion of urate, the salts of uric acid.[2] Renal under excretion of uric acid is the primary cause of hyperuricemia in about 90% of cases, while overproduction is the cause in less than 10%. About 10% of people with hyperuricemia develop gout at some point in their lifetimes. The risk, however, varies depending on the degree of hyperuricemia. When levels are between 415 and 530 μmol/L (7 and 8.9 mg/dL), the risk is 0.5% per year, while in those with a level greater than 535 μmol/L (9 mg/dL), the risk is 4 5% per year.

Lifestyle

Dietary causes account for about 12% of gout, and include a strong association with the consumption of alcohol, fructose-sweetened drinks, meat, and seafood. Other triggers include physical trauma and surgery. Recent studies have found dietary factors once believed to be associated are in fact not, including the intake of purine-rich vegetables and total protein. Coffee, vitamin C and dairy products consumption and physical fitness appear to decrease the risk. This is believed to be partly due to their effect in reducing insulin resistance.

Genetics

The occurrence of gout is partly genetic, contributing to about 60% of variability in uric acid level. A few rare genetic disorders, including familial juvenile hyperuricemic nephropathy, medullary cystic kidney disease, phosphoribosylpyrophosphate synthetase superactivity, and hypoxanthine-guanine phosphoribosyltransferase deficiency as seen in Lesch-Nyhan syndrome, are complicated by gout.

Medical conditions

Gout frequently occurs in combination with other medical problems. Metabolic syndrome, a combination of abdominal obesity, hypertension, insulin resistance and abnormal lipid levels occurs in nearly 75% of cases. Other conditions which are commonly complicated by gout include: polycythemia, lead poisoning, renal failure, hemolytic anemia, psoriasis, and solid organ transplants. A body mass index greater than or equal to 35 increases a male's risk of gout threefold. Chronic lead exposure and lead-contaminated alcohol are risk factors for gout due to the harmful effect of lead on kidney function. Lesch-Nyhan syndrome is often associated with gouty arthritis.

Medication

Diuretics have been associated with attacks of gout. However, a low dose of hydrochlorothiazide does not seem to increase the risk. Other medicines that have been associated include niacin and aspirin (acetylsalicylic acid). Cyclosporine is also associated with gout, particularly when used in combination with hydrochlorothiazide, as are the immunosuppressive drugs ciclosporin and tacrolimus.

Diagnosis

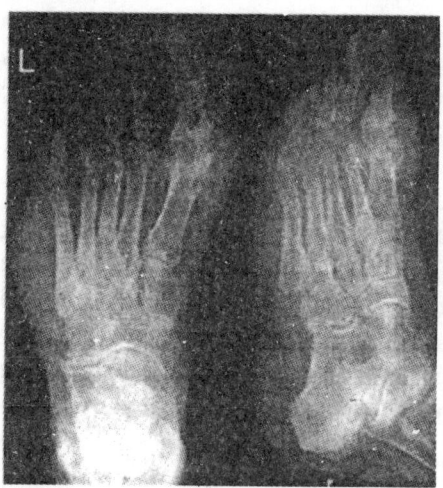

**Fig.2. Gout on X-ray of a left foot.
Typical location at the big toe joint.**

Gout may be diagnosed and treated without further investigations in someone with hyperuricemia and the classic podagra. Synovial fluid analysis should be done, however, if the diagnosis is in doubt. X-rays, while useful for identifying chronic gout, have little utility in acute attacks.

Synovial fluid

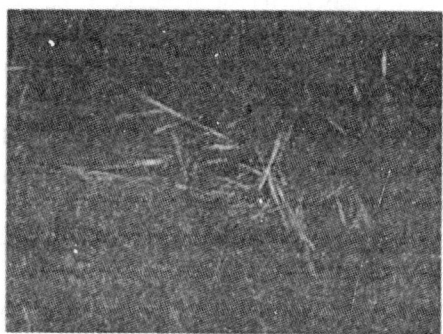

Fig.3. Formation of uric acid crystals in the joints is associated with gout.

A definitive diagnosis of gout is based upon the identification of monosodium urate (MSU) crystals in synovial fluid or a tophus. All synovial fluid samples obtained from undiagnosed inflamed joints should be examined for these crystals. Under polarized light microscopy, they have a needle-like morphology and strong negative birefringence. This test is difficult to perform, and often requires a trained observer. The fluid must also be examined relatively quickly after aspiration, as temperature and pH affect their solubility.

Blood tests

Hyperuricemia is a classic feature of gout; gout occurs, however, nearly half of the time without hyperuricemia, and most people with raised uric acid levels never develop gout. Thus, the diagnostic utility of measuring uric acid level is limited. Hyperuricemia is defined as a plasma urate level greater than 420 µmol/L (7.0 mg/dL) in males and 360 µmol/L (6.0 mg/dL) in females. Other blood tests commonly performed are white blood cell count, electrolytes, renal function, and erythrocyte sedimentation rate (ESR). However, both the white blood cells and ESR may be elevated due to gout in the absence of infection. A white blood cell count as high as 4.0×10^9/L (40,000/mm^3) has been documented.

Differential diagnosis

The most important differential diagnosis in gout is septic arthritis. This should be considered in those with signs of infection or those who do not improve with treatment. To help with diagnosis, a synovial fluid Gram stain and culture may be performed. Other conditions which present similarly include pseudogout and rheumatoid arthritis. Gouty tophi, in particular when not located in a joint, can be mistaken for basal cell carcinoma, or other neoplasms.

Treatment

The initial aim of treatment is to settle the symptoms of an acute attack. Repeated attacks can be prevented by different drugs used to reduce the serum uric acid levels. Ice applied for 20 to 30 minutes several times a day decreases pain. Options for acute treatment include nonsteroidal anti-inflammatory drugs (NSAIDs), colchicine and steroids, while options for prevention include allopurinol, probenecid and febuxostat. Lowering uric acid levels can cure the disease. Treatment of comorbidities is also important.

NSAIDs

NSAIDs are the usual first-line treatment for gout, and no specific agent is significantly more or less effective than any other. Improvement may be seen within 4 hours, and treatment is recommended for 1-2 weeks. They are not recommended, however in those with certain other health problems, such as gastrointestinal bleeding, renal failure, or heart failure. While indomethacin has historically been the most commonly used NSAID, an alternative, such as ibuprofen, may be preferred due to its better side effect profile in the absence of superior effectiveness. For those at risk of gastric side effects from NSAIDs, an additional proton pump inhibitor may be given.

Colchicine

Colchicine is an alternative for those unable to tolerate NSAIDs. Its side effects (primarily gastrointestinal upset) limit its usage. Gastrointestinal upset, however, depends on the dose, and the risk can be decreased by using smaller yet still effective doses. Colchicine may interact with other commonly prescribed drugs, such as atorvastatin and erythromycin, among others.

Steroids

Glucocorticoids have been found to be as effective as NSAIDs and may be used if contraindications exist for NSAIDs. They also lead to improvement when injected into the joint; the risk of a joint infection must be excluded, however, as they worsen this condition.

Pegloticase

Pegloticase (Krystexxa) was approved to treat gout in 2010. It will be an option for the 3% of people who are not adequately treated with other medications due to their association with severe allergic reactions. Pegloticase is administered as an intravenous infusion every two weeks. As of March 2010, however, no double blind, placebo controlled trials have been completed.

Prophylaxis

A number of medications are useful for preventing further episodes of gout, including allopurinol, probenecid, and febuxostat. They are not usually commenced until one to two weeks after an acute attack has resolved, due to theoretical concerns of worsening the attack, and are often used in combination with either an NSAID or colchicine for the first 3-6 months. They are not recommended until a person has suffered two attacks of gout, unless destructive joint changes, tophi, or urate nephropathy exist, as it is not until this point that medications have been found to be cost effective. Urate-lowering measures should be increased until serum uric acid levels are below 300-360 µmol/L (5.0-6.0 mg/dL) and are continued indefinitely. If these medications are being used chronically at the time of an attack, it is recommended they be continued.

Allopurinol blocks uric acid production, and is the most commonly used hypourecemic agent. Long term therapy is safe and well tolerated, and can be used in people with renal impairment or urate stones, although hypersensitivity occurs in a small number of individuals. Probenecid is effective for treating hyperuricemia, but has been found to be less effective than allopurinol. Febuxostat, a nonpurine inhibitor of xanthine oxidase, is now available as an alternative to allopurinol. It is approved in both Europe and the United States.

PART C NEOPLASTIC DISEASES

6.5 ACUTE LEUKAEMIAS

Leukemia or Leukaemia is a type of cancer of the blood or bone marrow that is characterized by an abnormal increase of white blood cells. Leukemia is a broad term covering a spectrum of diseases. In turn, it is part of the even broader group of diseases called hematological neoplasms.

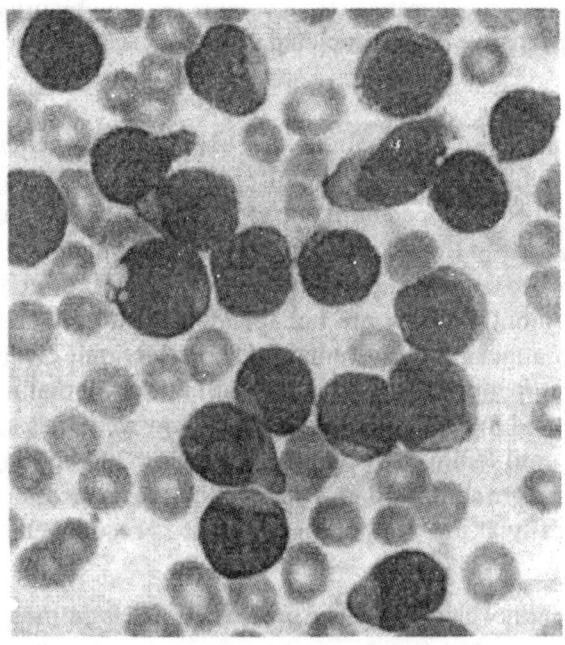

Fig.4. A Wright's stained bone marrow aspirate smear of patient with precursor B-cell acute lymphoblastic leukemia.

CLASSIFICATION

Four major kinds of leukemia

Cell type	Acute	Chronic
Lymphocytic leukemia (or "lymphoblastic")	Acute lymphoblastic leukemia (ALL)	Chronic lymphocytic leukemia (CLL)
Myelogenous leukemia (also "myeloid" or "nonlymphocytic")	Acute myelogenous leukemia (AML)	Chronic myelogenous leukemia (CML)

Leukemia is clinically and pathologically subdivided into a variety of large groups. The first division is between its *acute* and *chronic* forms:

- **Acute leukemia** is characterized by the rapid increase of immature blood cells. This crowding makes the bone marrow unable to produce healthy blood cells. Immediate treatment is required in acute leukemia due to the rapid progression and accumulation of the malignant cells, which then spill over into the bloodstream and spread to other organs of the body. Acute forms of leukemia are the most common forms of leukemia in children.

- **Chronic leukemia** is distinguished by the excessive build up of relatively mature, but still abnormal, white blood cells. Typically taking months or years to progress, the cells are produced at a much higher rate than normal cells, resulting in many abnormal white blood cells in the blood. Whereas acute leukemia must be treated immediately, chronic forms are sometimes monitored for some time before treatment to ensure maximum effectiveness of therapy. Chronic leukemia mostly occurs in older people, but can theoretically occur in any age group.

Additionally, the diseases are subdivided according to which kind of blood cell is affected. This split divides leukemias into lymphoblastic or *lymphocytic* and myeloid or *myelogenous leukemias*:

- In lymphoblastic or **lymphocytic leukemias**, the cancerous change takes place in a type of marrow cell that normally goes on to form lymphocytes, which are infection-fighting immune system cells. Most lymphocytic leukemias involve a specific subtype of lymphocyte, the B cell.

- In myeloid or **myelogenous leukemias**, the cancerous change takes place in a type of marrow cell that normally goes on to form red blood cells, some other types of white cells, and platelets.

    Combining these two classifications provides a total of four main categories. Within these main categories, there are typically several subcategories. Finally, some rarer types are usually considered to be outside of this classification scheme.

- **Acute lymphoblastic leukemia** (ALL) is the most common type of leukemia in young children. This disease also affects adults, especially those ages 65 and older. Standard treatments involve chemotherapy and radiation. The survival rates vary by age: 85% in children and 50% in adults. Subtypes include precursor B acute lymphoblastic leukemia, precursor T acute lymphoblastic leukemia, Burkitt's leukemia, and acute biphenotypic leukemia.

- **Chronic lymphocytic leukemia** (CLL) most often affects adults over the age of 55. It sometimes occurs in younger adults, but it almost never affects children. Two-thirds of affected people are men. The five-year survival rate is 75%. It is incurable, but there are many effective treatments. One subtype is B-cell prolymphocytic leukemia, a more aggressive disease.

- **Acute myelogenous leukemia** (AML) occurs more commonly in adults than in children, and more commonly in men than women. AML is treated with chemotherapy. The five-year survival rate is 40%. Subtypes of AML include acute promyelocytic leukemia, acute myeloblastic leukemia, and acute megakaryoblastic leukemia.

- **Chronic myelogenous leukemia** (CML) occurs mainly in adults. A very small number of children also develop this disease.

Treatment is with imatinib (Gleevec) or other drugs. The five-year survival rate is 90%. One subtype is chronic monocytic leukemia.

- **Hairy cell leukemia** (HCL) is sometimes considered a subset of CLL, but does not fit neatly into this pattern. About 80% of affected people are adult men. There are no reported cases in young children. HCL is incurable, but easily treatable. Survival is 96% to 100% at ten years.

- **T-cell prolymphocytic leukemia** (T-PLL) is a very rare and aggressive leukemia affecting adults; somewhat more men than women are diagnosed with this disease. Despite its overall rarity, it is also the most common type of mature T cell leukemia; nearly all other leukemias involve B cells. It is difficult to treat, and the median survival is measured in months.

- **Large granular lymphocytic leukemia** may involve either T-cells or NK cells; like hairy cell leukemia, which involves solely B cells, it is a rare and indolent (not aggressive) leukemia.

- **Adult T-cell leukemia** is caused by human T-lymphotropic virus (HTLV), a virus similar to HIV. Like HIV, HTLV infects CD4+ T-cells and replicates within them; however, unlike HIV, it does not destroy them. Instead, HTLV "immortalizes" the infected T-cells, giving them the ability to proliferate abnormally.

SIGNS AND SYMPTOMS

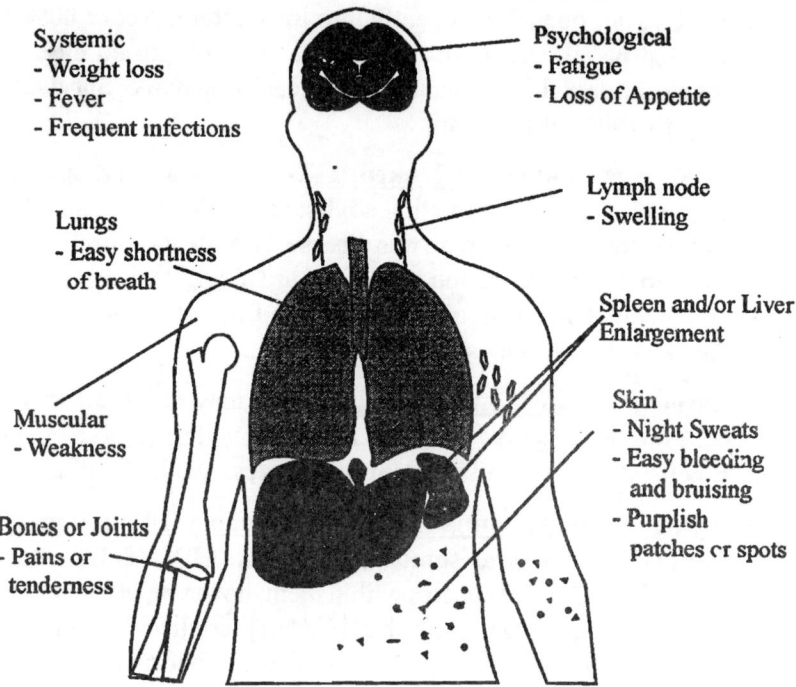

Fig.5. Common symptoms of chronic or acute leukemia

Damage to the bone marrow, by way of displacing the normal bone marrow cells with higher numbers of immature white blood cells, results in a lack of blood platelets, which are important in the blood clotting process. This means people with leukemia may easily become bruised, bleed excessively, or develop pinprick bleeds (petechiae).

White blood cells, which are involved in fighting pathogens, may be suppressed or dysfunctional. This could cause the patient's immune system to be unable to fight off a simple infection or to start attacking other body cells. Because leukemia prevents the immune system from working normally, some patients experience frequent infection, ranging from infected tonsils, sores in the mouth, or diarrhea to life-threatening pneumonia or opportunistic infections.

Finally, the red blood cell deficiency leads to anemia, which may cause dyspnea and pallor.

Some patients experience other symptoms. These symptoms might include feeling sick, such as having fevers, chills, night sweats and other flu-like symptoms, or feeling fatigued. Some patients experience nausea or a feeling of fullness due to an enlarged liver and spleen; this can result in unintentional weight loss. If the leukemic cells invade the central nervous system, then neurological symptoms (notably headaches) can occur.

All symptoms associated with leukemia can be attributed to other diseases. Consequently, leukemia is always diagnosed through medical tests.

The word *leukemia*, which means 'white blood', is derived from the disease's namesake high white blood cell counts that most leukemia patients have before treatment. The high numbers of white blood cells are apparent when a blood sample is viewed under a microscope. Frequently, these extra white blood cells are immature or dysfunctional. The excessive number of cells can also interfere with the level of other cells, causing a harmful imbalance in the blood count.

Some leukemia patients do not have high white blood cell counts visible during a regular blood count. This less-common condition is called *Aleukemia*. The bone marrow still contains cancerous white blood cells which disrupt the normal production of blood cells, but they remain in the marrow instead of entering the bloodstream, where they would be visible in a blood test. For an aleukemic patient, the white blood cell counts in the bloodstream can be normal or low. Aleukemia can occur in any of the four major types of leukemia, and is particularly common in hairy cell leukemia.

CAUSES

No single known cause for all of the different types of leukemia exists. The known causes, which are not generally factors within the control of the average person, account for relatively few cases. The different leukemias likely have different causes.

Leukemia, like other cancers, results from somatic mutations in the DNA. Certain mutations produce leukemia by activating oncogenes or deactivating tumor suppressor genes, and thereby disrupting the regulation of cell death, differentiation or division. These mutations may occur spontaneously or as a result of exposure to radiation or carcinogenic substances, and are likely to be influenced by genetic factors.

Among adults, the known causes are natural and artificial ionizing radiation, a few viruses such as Human T-lymphotropic virus, and some chemicals, notably benzene and alkylating chemotherapy agents for previous malignancies. Use of tobacco is associated with a small increase in the risk of developing acute myeloid leukemia in adults. Cohort and case-control studies have linked exposure to some petrochemicals and hair dyes to the development of some forms of leukemia. A few cases of maternal-fetal transmission have been reported. Diet has very limited or no effect, although eating more vegetables may confer a small protective benefit.

Viruses have also been linked to some forms of leukemia. Experiments on mice and other mammals have demonstrated the relevance of retroviruses in leukemia, and human retroviruses have also been identified. The first human retrovirus identified was Human T-lymphotropic virus, or HTLV-1, is known to cause adult T-cell leukemia.

Some people have a genetic predisposition towards developing leukemia. This predisposition is demonstrated by family histories and twin studies. The affected people may have a single gene or multiple genes in common. In some cases, families tend to develop the same kind of leukemia as other members; in other families, affected people may develop different forms of leukemia or related blood cancers.

In addition to these genetic issues, people with chromosomal abnormalities or certain other genetic conditions have a greater risk of leukemia. For example, people with Down syndrome have a significantly increased risk of developing forms of acute leukemia, and Fanconi anemia is a risk factor for developing acute myeloid leukemia.

Whether non-ionizing radiation causes leukemia has been studied for several decades. The International Agency for Research on Cancer expert working group undertook a detailed review of all data on static and extremely low frequency electromagnetic energy, which occurs naturally and in association with the generation, transmission, and use of electrical power. They concluded that there is limited evidence that high levels of ELF magnetic (but not electric) fields might cause childhood leukemia. Exposure to significant ELF magnetic fields might result in twofold excess risk for leukemia for children exposed to these high levels of magnetic fields. However, the report also says that methodological weaknesses and biases in these studies have likely caused the risk to be overstated. No evidence for a relationship to leukemia or another form of malignancy in adults has been demonstrated. Since exposure to such levels of ELFs is relatively uncommon, the World Health Organization concludes that ELF exposure, if later proven to be causative, would account for just 100 to 2400 cases worldwide each year, representing 0.2 to 4.9% of the total incidence of childhood leukemia for that year (about 0.03 to 0.9% of all leukemias).

DIAGNOSIS

Diagnosis is usually based on repeated complete blood counts and a bone marrow examination following symptoms observed. A lymph node biopsy can be performed as well in order to diagnose certain types of leukemia in certain situations. Following diagnosis, blood chemistry tests can be used to determine the degree of liver and kidney damage or the effects of chemotherapy on the patient. When concerns arise about visible damage due to leukemia, doctors may use an X-ray, MRI, or ultrasound. These can potentially view leukemia's effects on such body parts as bones (X-ray), the brain (MRI), or the kidneys, spleen, and liver (ultrasound). Finally, CT scans are rarely used to check lymph nodes in the chest.

Despite the use of these methods to diagnose whether or not a patient has leukemia, many people have not been diagnosed because many of the symptoms are vague, unspecific, and can refer to other diseases. For this reason, the American Cancer Society predicts that at least one-fifth of the people with leukemia have not yet been diagnosed.

TREATMENT

Most forms of leukemia are treated with pharmaceutical medications, typically combined into a multi-drug chemotherapy regimen. Some are also treated with radiation therapy. In some cases, a bone marrow transplant is useful.

Acute lymphoblastic leukemia

Management of ALL focuses on control of bone marrow and systemic (whole-body) disease. Additionally, treatment must prevent leukemic cells from spreading to other sites, particularly the central nervous system (CNS) e.g. monthly lumbar punctures. In general, ALL treatment is divided into several phases:

- **Induction chemotherapy** to bring about bone marrow remission. For adults, standard induction plans include prednisone, vincristine, and an anthracycline drug; other drug plans may include L-asparaginase or cyclophosphamide. For children with low-risk ALL, standard therapy usually consists of three drugs (prednisone, L-asparaginase, and vincristine) for the first month of treatment.

- **Consolidation therapy or intensification therapy** to eliminate any remaining leukemia cells. There are many different approaches to consolidation, but it is typically a high dose, multi-drug treatment that is undertaken for a few months. Patients with low to average risk ALL receive therapy with antimetabolite drugs such as methotrexate and 6 mercaptopurine (6-MP). High-risk patients receive higher drug doses of these drugs, plus additional drugs.

- **CNS prophylaxis** (preventive therapy) to stop the cancer from spreading to the brain and nervous system in high-risk patients. Standard prophylaxis may include radiation of the head and/or drugs delivered directly into the spine.

- **Maintenance treatments** with chemotherapeutic drugs to prevent disease recurrence once remission has been achieved. Maintenance therapy usually involves lower drug doses, and may continue for up to three years.

- Alternatively, **allogeneic bone marrow transplantation** may be appropriate for high-risk or relapsed patients.

Chronic lymphocytic leukemia

Decision to treat

Hematologists base CLL treatment on both the stage and symptoms of the individual patient. A large group of CLL patients have low-grade disease, which does not benefit from treatment. Individuals with CLL-related complications or more advanced disease often benefit from treatment. In general, the indications for treatment are:

- Falling hemoglobin or platelet count

- Progression to a later stage of disease

- Painful, disease-related overgrowth of lymph nodes or spleen

- An increase in the rate of lymphocyte production

Typical treatment approach

CLL is probably incurable by present treatments. The primary chemotherapeutic plan is combination chemotherapy with chlorambucil or cyclophosphamide, plus a corticosteroid such as prednisone or prednisolone. The use of a corticosteroid has the additional benefit of suppressing some related autoimmune diseases, such as immunohemolytic anemia or immune-mediated thrombocytopenia. In resistant cases, single-agent treatments with nucleoside drugs such as fludarabinea, pentostatin, or cladribine may be successful. Younger patients may consider allogeneic or autologous bone marrow transplantation.

Acute myelogenous leukemia

Many different anti-cancer drugs are effective for the treatment of AML. Treatments vary somewhat according to the age of the patient and according to the specific subtype of AML. Overall, the strategy is to control bone marrow and systemic (whole-body) disease, while offering specific treatment for the central nervous system (CNS), if involved.

In general, most oncologists rely on combinations of drugs for the initial, *induction phase* of chemotherapy. Such combination chemotherapy usually offers the benefits of early remission and a lower risk of disease resistance. *Consolidation* and *maintenance* treatments are intended to prevent disease recurrence. Consolidation treatment often entails a repetition of induction chemotherapy or the intensification chemotherapy with additional drugs. By contrast, maintenance treatment involves drug doses that are lower than those administered during the induction phase.

Chronic myelogenous leukemia

There are many possible treatments for CML, but the standard of care for newly diagnosed patients is imatinib (Gleevec) therapy. Compared to most anti-cancer drugs, it has relatively few side effects and can be taken orally at home. With this drug, more than 90% of patients will be able to keep the disease in check for at least five years, so that CML becomes a chronic, manageable condition.

In a more advanced, uncontrolled state, when the patient cannot tolerate imatinib, or if the patient wishes to attempt a permanent cure, then an allogeneic bone marrow transplantation may be performed. This procedure involves high-dose chemotherapy and radiation followed by infusion of bone marrow from a compatible donor. Approximately 30% of patients die from this procedure.

Hairy cell leukemia

Decision to treat

Patients with hairy cell leukemia who are symptom-free typically do not receive immediate treatment. Treatment is generally considered necessary when the patient shows signs and symptoms such as low blood cell counts (e.g., infection-fighting neutrophil count below 1.0 K/uL), frequent infections, unexplained bruises, anemia, or fatigue that is significant enough to disrupt the patient's everyday life.

Typical treatment approach

Patients who need treatment usually receive either one week of cladribine, given daily by intravenous infusion or a simple injection under the skin, or six months of pentostatin, given every four weeks by intravenous infusion. In most cases, one round of treatment will produce a prolonged remission.

Other treatments include rituximab infusion or self-injection with Interferon-alpha. In limited cases, the patient may benefit from *splenectomy* (removal of the spleen). These treatments are not typically given as the first treatment because their success rates are lower than cladribine or pentostatin.

T-cell prolymphocytic leukemia

Most patients with T-cell prolymphocytic leukemia, a rare and aggressive leukemia with a median survival of less than one year, require immediate treatment.

T-cell prolymphocytic leukemia is difficult to treat, and it does not respond to most available chemotherapeutic drugs. Many different treatments have been attempted, with limited success in certain patients: purine   analogues (pentostatin,   fludarabine, cladribine),chlorambucil, and various forms of combination chemotherapy (cyclophosphamide, doxorubicin, vincristine, prednisone CHOP, cyclophosphamide, vincristine, prednisone [COP], vincristine, doxorubicin, prednisone, etoposide, cyclophosphamide, bleomycin VAPEC-B). Alemtuzumab (Campath), a monoclonal antibody that attacks white blood cells, has been used in treatment with greater success than previous options.

Some patients who successfully respond to treatment also undergo stem cell transplantation to consolidate the response.

Juvenile myelomonocytic leukemia

Treatment for juvenile myelomonocytic leukemia can include splenectomy, chemotherapy, and bone marrow transplantation.

6.6 HODGKIN'S DISEASE

Hodgkin's disease is a type of lymphoma, a general name for a group of cancers of the blood that originate in the lymph glands. The lymph glands are organs of the immune system and are a part of the body's defense against infection and disease. Lymph glands are located throughout the body.

Hodgkin's disease, also called Hodgkin lymphoma, is the result of change or mutation in infection-fighting white blood cells called lymphocytes, which are stored in the lymph glands. This change results in an uncontrolled growth of cancer cells, which develop into malignant tumors in the lymph glands. Hodgkin's disease can also develop in other parts of the lymphatic system, such as the spleen or bone marrow.

TYPES OF HODGKIN'S DISEASE

There are two major types of Hodgkin's disease: Classical Hodgkins lymphoma and nodular lymphocyte-predominant Hodgkins disease.

Classical Hodgkin's Lymphoma: Classical Hodgkins lymphoma accounts for about 95% of Hodgkins disease cases. It has four major subtypes:

- **Nodular Sclerosis:** Nodular sclerosis is the most common subtype, representing about 60 - 80% of HD cases. Younger patients are more likely to have this type. The nodes first affected are often those located in the center of the chest (the mediastinum) or the neck.

- **Mixed Cellularity:** Mixed cellularity is the next most common HD form, occurring in about 15 - 30% of patients, mostly in older adults. Mixed cellularity refers to the presence of Reed-Sternberg cells and other cell types.

- **Lymphocyte Rich:** The lymphocyte-rich subtype accounts for about 5% of all HD cases. It tends to affect men more than women.

- **Lymphocyte Depleted:** The lymphocyte-depleted subtype is the least common type of HD, occurring in only about 1% of cases. It is usually seen in older people and patients infected with HIV. It is also more common in less developed countries. The cancer tends to be diagnosed when it is widespread, affecting the spleen, bone marrow, and liver as well as abdominal lymph nodes.

Nodular · Lymphocyte-Predominant Hodgkin's Disease: Nodular lymphocyte-predominant Hodgkin's disease occurs in about 5% of patients. It is distinct from classical Hodgkins lymphoma. The cells look like and are referred to as popcorn cells, which are variants of Reed-Sternberg cells. This type of HD typically affects younger patients and usually originates in the neck lymph nodes. This type of HD is sometimes confused with non-Hodgkins lymphoma (NHL). In fact, there is a 3 - 5% risk that nodular lymphocyte-predominant Hodgkins disease can transform into diffuse large B-cell NHL.

CAUSES, INCIDENCE, AND RISK FACTORS

The first sign of this cancer is often an enlarged lymph node which appears without a known cause. The disease can spread to nearby lymph nodes. Later it may spread to the spleen, liver, bone marrow, or other organs.

The cause is not known. Hodgkin's lymphoma is most common among people ages 15 - 35 and 50 - 70. Infection with the Epstein-Barr virus (EBV) is thought to contribute to most cases.

SIGNS AND SYMPTOMS

Patients with Hodgkin's lymphoma may present with the following symptoms:

- Night Sweats

- Unexplained weight loss

- Lymph nodes: the most common symptom of Hodgkin's is the painless enlargement of one or more lymph nodes. The nodes may also feel rubbery and swollen when examined. The nodes of the neck and shoulders (cervical and supraclavicular) are most frequently involved (80–90% of the time, on average). The lymph nodes of the chest are often affected, and these may be noticed on a chest radiograph.

- Splenomegaly: enlargement of the spleen occurs in about 30% of people with Hodgkin's lymphoma. The enlargement, however, is seldom massive and the size of the spleen may fluctuate during the course of treatment.

- Hepatomegaly: enlargement of the liver, due to liver involvement, is present in about 5% of cases.

- Hepatosplenomegaly: the enlargement of both the liver and spleen caused by the same disease.

- Pain

- Pain following alcohol consumption: classically, involved nodes are painful after alcohol consumption, though this phenomenon is very uncommon.

- Back pain: nonspecific back pain (pain that cannot be localized or its cause determined by examination or scanning techniques) has been reported in some cases of Hodgkin's lymphoma. The lower back is most often affected.

- Red-colored patches on the skin, easy bleeding and petechiae due to low platelet count (as a result of bone marrow infiltration, increased trapping in the spleen etc. i.e. decreased production, increased removal)

- Systemic symptoms: about one-third of patients with Hodgkin's disease may also present with systemic symptoms, including low-grade fever; night sweats; unexplained weight loss of at least 10% of the patient's total body mass in six months or less, itchy skin (pruritus) due to increased levels of eosinophils in the bloodstream; or fatigue (lassitude). Systemic symptoms such as fever, night sweats, and weight loss are known as B symptoms; thus, presence of fever, weight loss, and night sweats indicate that the patient's stage is, for example, 2B instead of 2A.

- Cyclical fever: patients may also present with a cyclical high-grade fever known as the Pel-Ebstein fever, or more simply "P-E fever". However, there is debate as to whether or not the P-E fever truly exists.

SIGNS AND TESTS

The disease may be diagnosed after:

- Biopsy of suspected tissue
- Bone marrow biopsy
- Lymph node biopsy
- Detection of Reed-Sternberg (Hodgkin's lymphoma) cells by biopsy from any site

A staging evaluation (tumor staging) may be done to determine how far the disease has spread. The following procedures may be done:

- Blood chemistry tests
- Bone marrow biopsy
- CT scans of the chest, abdomen, and pelvis
- PET scan
- Physical examination

In some cases, abdominal surgery to take a piece of the liver and remove the spleen may be needed. However, because the other tests are now so good at detecting the spread of Hodgkin's lymphoma, this surgery is usually unnecessary.

Hodgkin's lymphoma may change the results of the following tests:

- Angiotensin converting enzyme (ACE) levels
- Blood differential
- Bone marrow aspiration
- Cryoglobulins
- Ferritin
- Gallium scan

- Lymphocyte count

DIAGNOSIS

Hodgkin's lymphoma must be distinguished from non-cancerous causes of lymph node swelling (such as various infections) and from other types of cancer. Definitive diagnosis is by lymph node biopsy (usually excisional biopsy with microscopic examination). Blood tests are also performed to assess function of major organs and to assess safety for chemotherapy. Positron emission tomography (PET) is used to detect small deposits that do not show on CT scanning. PET scans are also useful in functional imaging (by using a radio labeled glucose to image tissues of high metabolism). In some cases a Gallium Scan may be used instead of a PET scan.

PATHOLOGY

Macroscopy

Affected lymph nodes (most often, laterocervical lymph nodes) are enlarged, but their shape is preserved because the capsule is not invaded. Usually, the cut surface is white-grey and uniform; in some histological subtypes (e.g. nodular sclerosis) a nodular aspect may appear.

A fibrin ring granuloma may be seen.

Microscopy

Microscopic examination of the lymph node biopsy reveals complete or partial effacement of the lymph node architecture by scattered large malignant cells known as Reed-Sternberg cells (RSC) (typical and variants) admixed within a reactive cell infiltrate composed of variable proportions of lymphocytes, histiocytes, eosinophils, and plasma cells. The Reed-Sternberg cells are identified as large often bi-nucleated cells with prominent nucleoli and an unusual CD45-, CD30+, CD15+/- immunophenotype. In approximately 50% of cases, the Reed-Sternberg cells are infected by the Epstein-Barr virus.

Characteristics of classic Reed-Sternberg cells include large size (20–50 micrometres), abundant, amphophilic, finely granular/

homogeneous cytoplasm; two mirror-image nuclei (owl eyes) each with an eosinophilic nucleolus and a thick nuclear membrane (chromatin is distributed at the cell periphery).

Variants:

- Hodgkin cell (atypical mononuclear RSC) is a variant of RS cell, which has the same characteristics, but is mononucleated.

- Lacunar RSC is large, with a single hyperlobated nucleus, multiple, small nucleoli and eosinophilic cytoplasm which is retracted around the nucleus, creating an empty space ("lacunae").

- Pleomorphic RSC has multiple irregular nuclei.

- "Popcorn" RSC (lympho-histiocytic variant) is a small cell, with a very lobulated nucleus, small nucleoli.

- "Mummy" RSC has a compact nucleus, no nucleolus and basophilic cytoplasm.

Hodgkin's lymphoma can be sub-classified by histological type. The cell histology in Hodgkin's lymphoma is not as important as it is in non-Hodgkin's lymphoma: the treatment and prognosis in classic Hodgkin's lymphoma usually depends on the stage of disease rather than the histotype.

Specific Drugs and Drug Combinations Used in Hodgkin's Disease

The standard chemotherapy regimens for Hodgkin's disease are ABVD and Stanford V.

ABVD consists of a 4-drug combination:

- Doxorubicin (Adriamycin)
- Bleomycin
- Vinblastine
- Dacarbazine

Stanford V consists of a 7-drug combination:

- Doxorubicin (Adriamycin)
- Mechlorethamine (nitrogen mustard)
- Vincristine
- Vinblastine
- Bleomycin
- Etoposide
- Prednisone

BEACOPP (bleomycin, etoposide, Adriamycin, cyclophosphamide, vincristine, procarbazine, and prednisone) is a chemotherapy regimen reserved for high-risk patients. This regimen is proving to be extremely effective, particularly in advanced stages, with studies reporting remission rates of over 95% in patients with advanced Hodgkin's. However, this regimen also increases the risk for developing secondary cancers such as leukemia. Patients who are treated with BEACOPP should receive long-term follow-up care to monitor for side effects from this therapy.

TREATMENT

The most important factor in Hodgkin's lymphoma treatment is the stage of the disease. The number and regions of lymph nodes affected and whether only one or both sides of your diaphragm are involved also are important considerations. Other factors affecting decisions about treating this disease include:

- Your age
- Your symptoms
- Whether you're pregnant
- Your overall health status

The goal of treatment is to destroy as many malignant cells as possible and bring the disease into remission. As many as 95 percent of people with stage I or stage II Hodgkin's lymphoma survive for five years or more with proper treatment. The five-year survival rate for those with widespread Hodgkin's lymphoma is about 60 to 70 percent, according to the American Cancer Society. But those numbers are based on people treated before 1990, so the outcome may be even more promising for people with more recent diagnosis and treatment.

Treatment options include:

Chemotherapy

When the disease progresses and involves more lymph nodes or other organs, chemotherapy is the preferred treatment. Chemotherapy uses specific drugs in combination to kill tumor cells. The drugs travel through your bloodstream and can reach nearly all areas of your body.

A major concern with chemotherapy is the possibility of long-term side effects and complications, such as heart damage, lung damage, liver damage, fertility problems and secondary cancers, such as leukemia.

Although severe effects aren't common, an ongoing effort is being made to find equally effective regimens with less toxicity. Drug regimens have been developed for Hodgkin's lymphomas that substantially diminish the likelihood of long-range, life-threatening complications, including acute leukemia, in people who have received multiple courses of chemotherapy and radiation therapy.

Chemotherapy regimens are commonly referred to by their initials, such as:

- **ABVD,** which consists of doxorubicin (Adriamycin), bleomycin, vinblastine and dacarbazine.

- **BEACOPP,** which consists of bleomycin, etoposide, doxorubicin, cyclophosphamide, vincristine, procarbazine and prednisone.

- **Stanford V,** which consists of doxorubicin, vinblastine, mechlorethamine, etoposide, vincristine, bleomycin and prednisone. Those taking this regimen are also treated with radiation therapy.

- **COPP/ABVD,** which consists of cyclophosphamide, vincristine, procarbazine, prednisone, doxorubicin, bleomycin, vinblastine and dacarbazine.

- **MOPP,** which consists of mechlorethamine, vincristine, procarbazine and prednisone.

ABVD is currently the preferred treatment. Some people at high risk may receive a more intensive treatment, such as BEACOPP.

Radiation

When the disease is confined to a limited area, radiation therapy may be the treatment of choice. With radiation therapy, high-energy X-rays are used to kill cancer cells. It's typical to radiate the affected lymph nodes and the next area of nodes where the disease might progress. The length of radiation treatment varies, depending on the stage of the disease. Radiation therapy may be used alone, but it is commonly used with chemotherapy. If you relapse after radiation therapy, chemotherapy becomes necessary.

Some forms of radiation therapy may increase your risk of heart disease, stroke, thyroid problems, infertility and other forms of cancer, such as breast or lung cancer. Radiation can also damage nearby healthy tissue. Most children with Hodgkin's lymphoma are treated with chemotherapy, but they may also receive low-dose radiation therapy.

Bone marrow or stem cell transplant

If the disease returns after treatment, you may need a bone marrow or stem cell transplant. For this procedure, your own bone marrow or stem cells (autologous) are removed and treated to kill cancerous cells. Then the marrow or stem cells are frozen and stored for safekeeping. Next you receive high-dose chemotherapy to destroy cancerous cells in your body. Finally your frozen marrow or stem cells are thawed and injected into your body through your veins.

REVIEW QUESTIONS

ESSAY QUESTIONS

1. What isGout? Classify the drugs used in treatment of Gout.
2. Describe the pharmacological actions of allopurinol and colchicin.
3. What is leukaemia? Enumerate the pharmacological actions of Vincrystine and Prednisolone.
4. Write short notes on HyperUricemia, Sickle cell anaemia.
5. Classify anti neoplastic agents. Explain the mechanism of action of any two classes.
6. Give the pharmacological actions of Methotrixate and Cyclophosphamide.
7. Classify different types of Anaemia and indicate appropriate therapy with their rationale.
8. Describe rheumatic diseases , Gout and their treatment.

SHORT ANSWER QUESTIONS

9. Write short note on Anaemias.
10. Describe the terms Leukaemia, Sickle cell anemia.
11. What is anaemia?
12. Illustrate the drugs used in the Hodgkins disease.
13. What are the reasons for Anaemia ?
14. What are the different forms of Anaemia?

Write about treatment involved in Anaemias

Chapter 7

THERAPEUTIC DRUG MONITORING

7.1 INTRODUCTION

Therapeutic drug monitoring (TDM) is the measurement of drugs and their active metabolites in patients receiving medications for the purpose of optimizing their therapeutic effect while minimizing adverse effects. The basic assumption of TDM is that the circulating concentration of a drug correlates better with pharmacological effect than does the dosage of the drug given to the patient. Therefore, there are a number of things to be considered in order for therapeutic drug monitoring to be effective and this article will briefly address some of these.

Before discussing the indications for therapeutic drug monitoring, it is essential to have an understanding of basic pharmacology. When a drug is administered to a patient, a number of things happen. First, the body must be able to take up the drug and distribute it to the target site of action. A change in the amount of drug or metabolite in various body compartments over time is determined by *pharmacokinetics*. Once at the target site the drug must produce the desired effect, usually through binding with specific receptors. The effect a drug has on the body is determined by *pharmacodynamics*.

Pharmacokinetics describes what happens when a drug is administered and is dependent on the extent and rate of Absorption, Distribution, Metabolism and Elimination (ADME). Typically, most drugs are administered orally and the amount absorbed (bioavailability) depends on a number of factors such as the formulation (fast acting vs. extended release), solubility and pK of the drug, co-administration of other drugs or food, and gastric emptying times. The drug is usually absorbed in the small intestine by passive diffusion. After the drug is absorbed it enters the hepatic portal system and is transported directly to the liver. In the liver the drug may be extensively metabolized by hepatic enzymes before reaching the general circulatory system. Once in circulation, the drug is distributed to various fluids and tissues. The volume of distribution (VD) of a drug describes the extent of distribution and is dependent on the solubility of the drug, rate of perfusion of the tissue, and the extent of protein binding. Further metabolism of the drug may occur in the liver or specific tissues and finally the drug and metabolites are excreted, usually in the urine or feces.

Pharmacodynamics describes the physiological effect of the drug and metabolites. This includes the desired therapeutic effect of the drug as well as unwanted side-effects. Pharmacodynamic variability can arise from differences in drug-receptor interaction and receptor response.

7.2 CRITERIA FOR THERAPEUTIC DRUG MONITORING

1.   Test Availability

Obviously, a test for the drug and active metabolites must exist in order to perform therapeutic drug monitoring. Most routine chemistry analyzers offer immunoassays for the more common therapeutic drugs. Some drugs require more specialized chromatographic techniques such as gas chromatography (GC) or liquid chromatography (LC). This type of equipment is not commonly found in most clinical laboratories. Therefore, monitoring for these drugs may require sending the sample to a reference laboratory for analysis. The turn-around time for these analyses must be quick enough to produce clinically meaningful results, especially if a change in dosage is required due to toxicity or adverse reaction.

2.   Narrow Safety Margin

As mentioned above, the basic assumption for TDM is that the concentration of drug circulating in the bloodstream correlates well with the pharmacological effect of the drug. The drug concentration usually also correlates with the toxicity of the drug.

The therapeutic range often describes the minimum concentration required for effective therapy and the maximum concentration permissible, above which there is a potential for toxicity. If the therapeutic range (window) is large, then the drug is considered to be safer since a larger dose of drug is required to produce toxicity. Many of the newer antiepileptic drugs (e.g. Lamotrigine) and serotonin selective reuptake inhibitors (e.g. Paxil, Zoloft) have a wide therapeutic range and therefore do not require therapeutic drug monitoring. Dosages can be titrated upward until the desired therapeutic effect is reached and tapered if clinical signs of toxicity are noted.

Drugs such as aminoglycosides, digoxin, theophylline, and lithium have a narrow therapeutic range. This means that there is a very limited range of drug concentration that will produce a therapeutic effect. Below this range the drug will be ineffective or partially effective and above which it will be toxic. Therefore, a drug or other therapeutic agent with a narrow therapeutic range (i.e. with little difference between toxic and therapeutic doses) may have its dosage adjusted according to measurements of the actual blood levels.

3.   Compliance

Therapeutic drug monitoring can be considered in patients that do not show an apparent clinical response to a drug despite being on a seemingly adequate dosage. If the measured drug concentration appears consistent with the dosage of the drug, then the patient may be considered a non-responder to therapy. If the measured concentrations are very low or not detected then the patient is either "non-compliant" or is an unusually "fast metaboliser".

4.   High pharmacokinetic variability

Inter-individual variation in drug absorption, metabolism, and excretion can produce a poor correlation between drug concentration and dosage. Pharmacokinetic variability between patients can arise from multiple factors:

- Age - large pharmacokinetic differences between neonates, children, adults and geriatric individuals.

- Gender - differences due to body fat composition.

- Pregnancy - for example, plasma drug levels of phenytoin and phenobarbitone tend to be reduced during pregnancy.

- Drug-drug interactions - co-administration of drugs which inhibit metabolism may lead to higher than expected concentrations and toxicity while co-administration of drugs that induce metabolic enzymes may reduce concentrations and lead to ineffectiveness.

- Genetic polymorphisms in drug metabolizing enzymes (pharmacogenetics) – certain individuals may have polymorphic enzymes which are inactive or partially active resulting in delayed clearance while others may have multiple gene copies encoding for the enzyme resulting in "fast" or "rapid" metabolism of the drug.

- Malabsorption - increased microfloral colonization, accelerated GI transit, delayed gastric emptying, bowel surgery may influence the amount of drug absorbed

- Liver disease – decreased metabolism

- Kidney disease – decreased renal clearance

- Cardiovascular disease – decreased perfusion

Therapeutic drug monitoring may be useful in establishing the initial individualized dosage for a given patient in the above situations. Once the dosage is established however, there may be no more need for continued TDM as long as the patient's clinical condition remains the same.

5.   Therapeutic effect difficult to monitor

If there is an obvious clinical effect of a medication then TDM is usually not necessary. For example, drugs that lower blood pressure can be monitored directly by measuring blood pressure. Anticoagulants are more effectively monitored by measuring INR. If there is no clear physiological response to monitor and a drug is being used prophylactically, e.g. anticonvulsants, antiarrhythmics, depression, asthma, or organ rejection, then TDM may be warranted. Seizure activity in a patient taking anticonvulsants may indicate low drug concentrations or toxicity. The decision to increase or decrease the dose is most efficiently made on the basis of the serum concentration.

7.3 CONSIDERATIONS FOR TDM

1.   Sample type

Serum or plasma samples are usually collected for TDM. Serum separator tubes should be avoided since lipophilic drugs can dissolve in the gel barrier. The use of oral fluid (saliva) for drug monitoring has received a great deal of attention. Measuring drugs in oral fluid is appealing because samples can be obtained non-invasively. There are however a number of limitations to using oral-fluid. The concentration of a drug in saliva is proportional to the concentration of the unbound drug rather than to the total of bound and unbound drug, usually measured in a plasma sample. Intuitively, this should be preferred since the free unbound fraction of the drug should represent the active amount of drug in the body. While most drugs passively diffuse into the oral fluid, some drugs are actively secreted. Some drugs may reduce production and flow of saliva and stimulation of saliva flow may alter pH and hence diffusion of the drug.

2.   Timing of Sample

An important part of therapeutic drug monitoring is the timing of the blood collection. When a drug is administered, the blood concentration increases until it reaches a peak and then the concentration begins to fall. The lowest concentration (trough) is usually just before the next dose. The time required for the serum concentration of a drug to decrease by 50% is called the half life of the drug. When a drug is administered in intervals approximately equal to its half-life, a steady state concentration will be achieved after 4-5 half-lives. For drugs with a long half-life, there is little difference between the steady state peak and trough concentrations. For drugs with a short half-life, the differences between the peak and trough concentrations can be significant and both are usually measured (i.e. aminoglycosides).

Drugs that are given intravenously require time to redistribute into the different body compartments. In general, intravenous medications can be sampled 30-60 minutes post administration. Digoxin however requires 6 hours for redistribution to occur.

3.   Interpretation

Drug concentration determinations must always be interpreted in the context of the clinical situation. For example, a concentration of digoxin that would normally be therapeutic could be toxic if the patient also has hypokalemia.

7.5 THERAPEUTIC DRUG MONITORING: THERAPEUTIC AND TOXIC RANGE

Drug Level	Use	Therapeutic Level	Toxic
Aceteminophen mg/ml	Analgesic, antipyretic	Depends on use	>250
Amikacin mg/ml	Antibiotic	12-25 mg/ml	>25
Aminophylline ng/ml	Bronchodilator	10-20 mg/ml	>20
Amitriptyline ng/ml	Antidepressant	120-150 ng/ml	>500
Carbamazepine mg/ml	Anticonvulsant	5-12 mg/ml	>12
Chloramphenicol mg/ml	Antibiotic	10-20 mg/ml	>25
Digoxin ng/ml	Cardiotonic	0.8-2.0 ng/ml	>2.4
Gentamicin	Antibiotic	4-12 mg/L	>12 mg/L
Lidocaine	Antiarrhythmic	1.5-5.0 mg/ml	>5 mg/ml
Lithium mEq/L	Antimanic	0.7-2.0 mEq/L	>2.0
Nortriptyline ng/ml	Antidepressant	50-150 ng/ml	>500

Continued on next page

Drug Level	Use	Therapeutic Level	Toxic
Phenobarbital mg/ml	Anticonvulsant	10-30 mg/ml	>40
Phenytoin mg/ml	Anticonvulsant	7-20 mg/ml	>30
Procainamide mg/ml	Antiarrhythmic	4-8 mg/ml	>16
Propranolol ng/ml	Antiarrhythmic	50-100 ng/ml	>150
Quinidine mg/ml	Antiarrhytmic	1-4 mg/ml	>10
Theophylline mg/ml	Bronchodilator	10-20 mg/ml	>20
Tobramycin mg/ml	Antibiotic	4-12 mg/ml	>12
Valproic acid mg/ml	Anticonvulsant	50-100 mg/ml	>100

REVIEW QUESTIONS

ESSAY QUESTIONS

1. Write about Therapeutic drug monitoring in Geriatrics.
2. Explain the Therapeutic Drug Monitoring in Paediatrics.
3. Write a short note on Therapeutic Drug Monitoring.
4. What is meant by Therapeutic Drug Monitoring? What are the objectives? What are the stages of Drug Monitoring?
5. What are the advantages of Therapeutic Drug Monitoring.
6. Describe the TDM of
   a) Daibetes Mellitus
   b) Ischaemic Heart Disease.

SHORT ANSWER QUESTIONS

7. What are the objectives of TDM?
8. What are the stages of Drug Monitoring?
9. Describe the TDM of Ischaemic Heart Disease.
10. What are the important points to be remembered for TDM?

Chapter 8

CONCEPT OF ESSENTIAL DRUGS AND RATIONAL DRUG USE

8.1 INTRODUCTION

India is a country with significant drug use, where more than 50,000 drug formulations are licensed for sale, where substandard and counterfeit drugs find their way into the market. The non-availability of quality essential drugs, excessive availability of unnecessary drugs is common in health facilities. About 30-35 per cent of the health budget at the centre and in the states is spent on medicines. The number having access to allopathic medicines in rural areas is only around 35 per cent. Accessible health services, qualified staff and availability of quality drugs are essential components of any health care system but drugs have special importance for various reasons.

With the limited resources at the disposal of health care facilities, it is important to improve the management of existing resources. Many more persons requiring medicines could be provided with good quality medicines with the same resource if drug management system improves. Drug management system consists of four components; Selection, Procurement, Distribution and Use. Through the use of these components the availability of quality medicines can be improved.

WHO in 1975, defined essential drugs as "Those considered to be of utmost importance and hence basic, indispensable and necessary for the health needs of the population. They should be available at all times, in the proper dosage forms, to all segments of society". The WHO model list of Essential Medicines prepared first time in 1977, and is updated every two years since then. In Alma Ata in 1978, the WHO/UNICEF conference on primary health care adopted the essential drugs concept as one of the basic tools to improve health care.

Essential medicines are those satisfy the priority health care needs of the population. They are selected with due regard to public health relevance, evidence on efficacy and safety, and comparative cost effectiveness.

Numerous studies have indicated the impact of concept of essential medicines on the availability and proper use of medicines within health care systems. The concept is more important and relevant in country like India.

Implementation of the concept of essential drugs by Government of Tamil Nadu and Delhi as early as in 1994 showed significant improvement in drug availability in government health care facilities under their jurisdiction. Exactly which medicines are regarded as essential remains a national, regional or local responsibility.

The selection process for inclusion in EDL is critical. Though EDL of WHO may be used in the first instances, it requires to be best developed for different levels of care.

The wastage of drugs by prescribers and users is common. The notion that if one drug is good, two are better and three ideal are perceived by general public. The quantities of drugs prescribed for a given illness are often far more than what is reasonably needed. Drugs are often prescribed when no drug is needed at all, because patients expect or demand a pill or injection or because prescribers are anxious to be seen as doing something. Worldwide more than 50 per cent of all medicines are prescribed, dispensed or sold inappropriately, while 50 per cent of the patients fail to take them correctly.

Rational Use of Drugs is defined as "Patients receiving medication appropriate to their clinical needs, in doses that meet their own individual requirement, for an adequate period of time and at the lowest cost to them and their community".

8.2 THE PROBLEM OF IRRATIONAL USE OF DRUGS

Irrational or non-rational use is the use of medicines in a way that is not compliant with rational use as defined above. World wide more than 50 % of all medicines are prescribed, dispensed, or sold inappropriately, while 50 % of patients fail to take them correctly. Moreover, about one-third of the world's population lacks access to essential medicines, common types of irrational drugs use are:

- The use of too many drugs per patient (polypharmacy);

- Inappropriate use of antimicrobials, often in inadequate dosage, for non-bacterial infections;

- Over-use of injections when oral formulations would be more appropriate;

- Failure to prescribe in accordance with clinical guidelines;

- Inappropriate self-medication, often of prescription only drugs.

Lack of access to drugs and inappropriate doses result in serious morbidity and mortality, particularly for childhood infections and chronic diseases, such as hypertension, diabetes, epilepsy and mental disorders.

Inappropriate use and over-use of drugs waste resources often out-of pocket payments by patients and result in significant patient harm in terms of poor patient out comes and adverse drug reactions.

Furthermore, over-use of antimicrobials is leading to increased anti-microbial resistance and non-sterile injections to the transmission of hepatitis, HIV/AIDS and other blood, borne diseases. Finally, irrational over-use of drugs can stimulate inappropriate patient demand, and lead to reduced access and attendance rates due to medicine stock-outs and loss of patient confidence in the health system.

8.3 ASSESSING THE PROBLEM OF IRRATIONAL USE

To address irrational use of medicines, prescribing, dispensing and patient use should be regularly monitored in terms of:

● **The types** of irrational use, so that strategies can be targeted towards changing specific problems;

● **The amount** of irrational use. So that the size of the problem is known and the impact of the strategies can be monitored;

● **The reasons** why medicines are used irrationally. So that appropriate, effective and feasible strategies can be chosen. People often have very rational reasons for using medicines irrationally. Causes of irrational use include lack of knowledge, skills or independent information. Unrestricted availability of medicines, overwork of health personnel, inappropriate promotion of medicines and profit motives from selling medicines.

In general, two broad types of data, **quantitative and qualitative,** are useful for identifying problems of inappropriate drug use and for learning about their underlying causes.

8.4 QUANTITATIVE METHODS

Quantitative data are very useful for finding out what behaviors are happening in a given situation, and how often they are happening. These data can therefore be used to identify specific problems or to measure the success of interventions to change these problems.

Table 1 lists some of the wide range of quantitative data sources that may be useful in different situations for learning about drug use practices. It is clear that there are many possible ways to measure different aspects of drug use.

Table 1: Sources of quantitative Data on drug use

LOCATION OF DATA	DATA SOURCES	USEFUL FOR STUDYING
Public Sector Administrative Offices, Medical Stores	RETROSPECTIVE: ●drug supply orders ●stock cards ●shipping and delivery receipts	●Aggregate patterns of drug use and expenditures ●Comparative use of drugs within therapeutic classes ●Comparative use by different facilities or areas

Continued on next page

LOCATION OF DATA	DATA SOURCES	USEFUL FOR STUDYING
Health Facility Clinical Treatment Areas and Medical Record Departments	RETROSPECTIVE •patient registers •health worker logs •pharmacy receipts •medical records PROSPECTIVE: •patient observations •patient exit surveys •inpatient surveys	•Aggregate patterns of drug use and expenditures •Drug use per case, overall & by group (age, sex, health problem, etc.) •Provider-specific prescribing patterns •Features of patient-prescriber interaction
Health Facility Pharmacies	RETROSPECTIVE •pharmacy logs •prescriptions retained in pharmacies PROSPECTIVE •patient exit surveys •patient observations	•Aggregate patterns of drug use and expenditures •Dispensing practices •features of patient dispenser interaction
Pharmacies and Retail Drug Outlets	RETROSPECTIVE •prescriptions retained in pharmacies PROSPECTIVE: •customer exit surveys •customer observations •"simulated visits"	•Private sector prescribing practices drug sales without prescription •Self-medication practices •Features of customer-sales attendant interaction
Households	RETROSPECTIVE: •family medical records •household surveys PROSPECTIVE •household drug audits •family medical records	•Total community drug use •Care-seeking behavior •Self-medication practices •Family drug use •Patient compliance

8.5 QUALITATIVE METHODS

Quantitative methods describe drug use patterns, or pinpoint specific problems that need attention. However, quantitative methods are usually not good for understanding *why* these patterns or problems exist. Qualitative techniques are better suited to examine underlying feelings, beliefs, attitudes, and motivations.

In order to change problems effectively, we often need to find out more about why they are happening. For this purpose, it is helpful to collect qualitative data about the problem in the form of descriptions, ratings, observations, or some other less easily quantifiable form.

Qualitative methods are based on talking to people, or observing their behavior.

Some common methods to collect qualitative data on drug use include; in-depth interviews, focus groups, structured observations, structured questionnaires, and simulated patient visits.

Experience from many countries has encouraged the development of a standard method of measuring drug use practices, based on drug use indicators.

WHO/INRUD have designed drug use indicator that can be used to identify general prescribing and quality of care problems at health care facilities since 1993.

8.6 SELECTED WHO/INRUD DRUG USE INDICATORS (WHO, 1993)

Prescribing indicators:

- % Medicines prescribed by generic name
- % Encounters with an antibiotic prescribed
- % Encounters with an injection prescribed
- % Medicines prescribed from essential medicines list or formulary

Patient care indicators:

• Average consultation time

• Average dispensing time

• % Medicines actually dispensed

• % Medicines adequately labeled

• % Patients with knowledge of correct doses

Facility indicators:

• Availability of essential drugs list or formulary to practitioners

• Availability of clinical guidelines

• % Key drugs available

Complementary Drug Use Indicators:

• Average drug cost per encounter

• % Prescriptions in accordance with clinical guidelines

Framework for Changing Drug Use Practices

A wide range of factors causes problems in drug use.

These factors differ in importance from problem to problem and from setting to setting. Before trying to correct any problem in drug use, it is helpful to identify which factors are most important in causing the problem at hand. These can be identified using the methods mentioned under the title assessing the problem of irrational use.

8.7 OVERVIEW OF INTERVENTION STRATEGIES

Different strategies can improve drug use. These strategies can be grouped into three broad categories.

Educational: Seeking to inform or persuade prescribers, dispensers, or patients to use drugs in a different way. .

Managerial: Structuring or guiding decisions through the use of specific processes, forms, packages, or monetary incentives.

Regulatory: restricting allowable decisions by placing absolute limits on availability of drugs.

As you consider each intervention think about the settings and types of problem for which it may be appropriate. Which of the possible underlying factors influencing drug use does each intervention target? What would the potential strengths and weaknesses of such a strategy be in your institution?

When thinking about interventions, remember that it is usually more effective to combine several different strategies to improve a single problem in drug use.

For example, in-service training programs for prescribers about malaria treatment can be combined with supportive community education through the media. Or regulations that limit access to anti-diarrhea drugs can be combined with the dissemination of standard diarrhea treatment guidelines.

8.8   WHO/INRUD RECOMMENDS *TWELVE CORE INTERVENTIONS* TO PROMOTE MORE RATIONAL USE OF DRUGS

1.   A mandate multi-disciplinary national body to coordinate medicine use policies

2.   Clinical guidelines

3.   Essential drugs list based on treatments of choice

4.   Drugs and Therapeutics Committees districts and hospitals

5.   Problem-based pharmacotherapy training in undergraduate curricula

6.   Continuing in-service medical education as a licensure requirement

7.   Supervision, audit and feedback

8.   Independent information on drugs

9.   Public education about drugs

10. Avoidance of perverse financial incentives

11. Appropriate and enforced regulation

12. Sufficient government expenditure to ensure availability of drugs and staff.

1.   A mandated multi-disciplinary national body to coordinate medicine use policies.

Many Societal and health system factors, as well as professionals and many others, contribute to how drugs are used. Therefore, a multi-disciplinary approach is needed to develop, implement and evaluate interventions to promote more rational use of medicines.

A national regulatory authority is important in materializing these activities. In case of our country, the Drug Administration and Control Authority (DACA) is the agency that develops and implements most of the legislation and regulation on pharmaceuticals. Ensuring rational use will require many additional activities, which will need coordination with many stakeholders.

Thus a national body is needed to coordinate policy and strategies at National level, in both the public and private sectors.

2.   Clinical guidelines

Clinical Guidelines (Standard treatment guidelines, prescribing policies) consists of systematically developed statements to help prescribers make decisions about appropriate treatments for specific clinical conditions. Evidence - based clinical guidelines are critical to promoting rational use of drugs. Firstly they provide a benchmark of satisfactory diagnosis and treatment against which comparison of actual treatments can be made. Secondly, they are a proven way to promote more rational use of drugs provided they are: (1) developed in a participatory way involving end-users, (2) easy to read; (3) introduced with an official launch, training and wide dissemination; and (4) reinforced by prescription audit and feedback. Guidelines should be developed for each level of care (ranging from paramedical staff in primary health care clinics to specialist doctors in tertiary referral hospitals), based on prevalent clinical conditions and the skills of available prescribers. Evidence-based treatment recommendations and regular updating help to ensure credibility and acceptance of the guidelines by practitioners. Sufficient resources are needed to reimburse all those who contribute to the guidelines, and to cover the costs of printing, dissemination and training.

Currently, Drug Administration and Control Authority (DACA) of Ethiopia have developed standard treatment guidelines for different health facilities including for zonal and District Hospitals, Health Centers and for Health stations. These guidelines are supposed to be disseminated in the near future to all health institutions in the country.

3.   Essential Drugs list based on treatments of choice

Essential drugs are those that satisfy the priority health care needs of the population.

Using an essential Drugs list (EDL) makes drugs management easier in all respects; procurement, storage and distribution are easier with fewer items; and prescribing and is dispensing are easier for professionals if they have to know about fewer items. A national EDL should be based upon national clinical guidelines. Drug selection should be done by a Central committee with an agreed membership and using explicit, previously agreed criteria, based on efficacy, safety, quality, cost (which will vary locally) and cost-effectiveness. EDLs should be regularly updated and their introduction accompanied by an official launch, training and dissemination. Public sector procurement and distribution of medicines should be limited primarily to those medicines on the EDL, and it must be ensured that only those health workers approved to use certain drugs are actually supplied with them. Government activities in the pharmaceutical sector (e.g. quality assurance, and training), should focus on the EDL. The Drug Administration and Control Authority (DACA) is currently developing EDL for Ethiopia using the WHO model list of Essential drugs as a starting point.

4.   Drugs and therapeutics committees in Hospitals

A Drugs and therapeutic committee (DTC) also called a pharmacy and therapeutics committee, is a committee designated to ensure the safe and effective use of medicines in the facility or area under its

Jurisdiction. Such committees are well established in industrial countries as a successful way of promoting more rational, cost-effective hospitals to have DTCs by making it an accreditation requirement to various professional societies. DTC members should represent all the major specialities and the administration; they should also be independent and declare any Conflict of interest. A senior doctor would usually be the chairperson and the chief pharmacist, the secretary. Factors critical to success include: clear objectives a firm mandate support by the senior hospital management; transparency, wide representation; technical competence; a multidisciplinary approach; and sufficient resources to implement the DTC's decisions.

Results of one study conducted a year before in Ethiopia revealed that only 44 % of the study group has already established DTC in their institutions but out of which less than 7 % were actively functional at study period.

The main functions of DTC are

• Evaluating and selecting drugs for the formulary and providing for its periodic revision. This includes developing rigorous evidence - based criteria for selection of drugs, taking into account efficacy, safety, quality and cost;

• Assessing drug use to identify potential problems.

• Promoting and conducting effective interventions to improve drug use (including educational, managerial and regulatory methods).

In addition Committees may;

• Manage adverse drug reactions

• Manage medication errors

• Promote infection control practices

5.   Problem-based training in pharmacotherapy in undergraduate curricula.

The quality of basic training in pharmacotherapy for undergraduate medical and paramedical students can significantly influence future prescribing. Rational pharmacotherapy training, linked to clinical guidelines and essential drugs lists, can help to establish good prescribing habits. Training is more successful if it is problem-based, concentrates on common clinical conditions, takes into account students' knowledge, attitudes and skills, and is targeted to the students' future prescribing requirements.

The guide to Good Prescribing describes the problem-based approach, which has been adopted in a number of medical schools.

6.   Continuing in-service medical education

Continuing in-service medical education (CME) is a requirement for licensure of health professionals in many industrialized countries. CME is likely to be more effective if it is problem based, targeted, involves professional societies, universities and the Ministry of Health, and is face- to -face. Printed materials that are unaccompanied by face-to-face interventions, have been found to be ineffective in changing prescribing or dispensing behavior. CME need not be limited only to professional medical or paramedical personnel, but may also include people in the informal sector such as medicine retailers often CME activities are heavily dependent on the support of pharmaceutical companies, as public funds are insufficient. This type of CME may not unbiased. Governments should therefore support efforts by University departments and national professional associations to give independent CME.

7.   Supervision, audit and feed back

Supervision is essential to ensure good quality of care. Supervision that is supportive, educational and face-to-face will be more effective and better accepted by prescribers than simple inspection and punishment. Effective forms of supervision include prescription audit and feedback, peer review and group processes. Prescription audit and feedback consists of analyzing prescription appropriateness and then giving feedback. Prescribers may be told how their prescribing compares with accepted guidelines or with that of their peers. Involving peers in audit and feedback (peer review) is particularly effective. In hospitals, such audit and feedback is known as drug use evaluation.

Group process approaches amongst prescribers consists of health professionals themselves identifying a medicine use problem and developing, implementing and evaluating a strategy to correct the problem. This process needs facilitation by a moderator or supervisor.

8.   Independent Drug Information

Often, the only information about medicines that practitioners receive is provided by the Pharmaceutical industry and may be biased. Provision of independent (unbiased) information is therefore essential. Drug information centers (DICs) and drug bulletins are two useful ways to disseminate such information. Both may be run by government or a University teaching hospital or a non-governmental organization, under the supervision of a trained health professional. Whoever runs the DIC or bulletin must (1) be independent of outside influences and discloses any financial or other conflict of interest, and (2) use evidence-based medicine and transparent deduction for all recommendations made.

In our country the Drug Information Division of Drug Administration and control Authority run this activity. The divisions produce and cascade current awareness drug information bulletin quarterly and currently the division has published Drugs formulary that provides independent information on drugs available at District Hospital and Health Center level.

9.   Public Education about medicines

Without sufficient knowledge about the risks and benefits of using medicines and when and how to use them, people will often not get the expected clinical outcomes and may suffer adverse effects. This is true for prescribed medicines, as well as medicines used without the advice by health professionals. Governments have a responsibility to ensure both the quality of medicines and the quality of the information about medicines available to consumers. This will require medicines available to consumers. This will require.

- Ensuring the over-the-counter drugs is sold with adequate labeling and instructions that are accurate, legible, and easily understood by lay persons. The information should include the medicine name, indications, contraindications, dosage, drug interactions and warnings concerning unsafe use or storage.

• Monitoring and regulating advertising, which may adversely influence consumers as well as prescribers, and which may occur through television, radio, newspapers and the internet.

• Running targeted Public education campaigns, which take into account cultural beliefs and the influence of social factors. Education about the use of medicines may be introduced into the health education component of school curricula or into adult education programs, such literacy courses.

10.   Avoidance of perverse financial incentives

Financial incentives may strongly promote rational or irrational use. For example, prescribers who earn money from the sale of medicines (e.g. dispensing doctors) prescribe more medicines, and more expensive medicines, than prescribers who don't; therefore the health system should be organized so that prescribers do not dispense or sell medicines.

11.   Appropriate and enforced Regulation

Regulation of the activities of all actors involved in the use of medicines is critical to ensuring rational use. If regulations are to have any effect, they must be enforced and the regulatory authority must be sufficiently funded and backed up by the judiciary.

Regulatory measures to support rational use

• Registration of medicines to ensure that only safe efficacious medicines of good quality are available in the market and those unsafe non-efficacious drugs are banned.

• Limiting prescription of drugs by level of prescriber, that includes limiting certain drugs to being available only with a prescription and not available over-the-counter.

• Setting educational standards for health professionals and developing and enforcing codes of conduct; this requi.es the cooperation of the professional societies and universities.

• Licensing of health professionals - doctors, nurses, paramedics to ensure that all practitioners have the necessary competence with regard to diagnosis, prescribing and dispensing.

• Licensing of drug out lets - retails shops, wholesalers - to ensure that oil supply outlets maintain the necessary stocking and dispensing standards.

• Monitoring and regulating medicine promotion to ensure that it is ethical and unbiased. All promotional claims should be reliable, accurate, truthful, informative, balanced, up-to-date, capable of substantiation and in good taste.

12.   Sufficient Government expenditure to ensure availability of drugs and staff.

Back of essential medicines leads to the use of non-essential drugs, and lack of appropriately trained personnel leads to irrational prescribing by untrained personnel. Furthermore, without sufficient competent personnel and finances, it is impossible to carry out any of the core components of a national program to promote rational use of drugs. Poor clinical out come, needless suffering and economic waste are sufficient reasons for large government investment.

Governments are responsible for investing the necessary funds to ensure that all public health facilities have sufficient, appropriately trained health professionals and enough essential drugs at affordable prices for all the population, with specific provisions for the poor and disadvantaged. Achieving this will require limiting government procurement and supply to essential medicines only, and investing in adequate training, supervision and health staff salaries.

SUMMARY

Rational use of drugs requires that patients receive medications appropriate to their clinical needs, in doses that meet their individual requirements, for an adequate period of time, and at the lowest cost to them and their community.

Irrational drug use occurs with polypharmacy, with the use of wrong or ineffective drugs, or with under use or incorrect use of effective drugs. These actions have an adverse impact on the quality of drug therapy and cost and may cause adverse reactions or negative psychosocial impacts.

A prescriber's lack of knowledge and experience is only one factor in irrational drug use. Other underlying factors can be found in the dispensing process, the patient or community, and the health system itself.

Strategies to address irrational drug use can be characterized as educational, managerial, or regulatory. Whichever method to change drug use is selected, the intervention is likely to contain the elements of focusing on key factors, targeting facilities with the worst practices, and using credible sources and communication channels. Personal contact (face-to-face meetings, for example) can sometimes be used to convey a limited number of key messages; these can be repeated and clarified using different media.

When implementing a strategy, the logical steps are to

• Identify the problem

• Understand the underlying causes;

• List possible interventions;

• Asses available resources;

• Choose an intervention;

• Monitor and restructure the activity, as necessary

Interventions should be based on an understanding of the cause of the problem and on active strategies to change behavior. Experience indicates that the most effective interventions are those that

• Identify key influence factors;

• Target individuals or groups with the worst practices;

• Use credible communication channels;

• Use personal contact whenever possible;

• Limit the number of messages;

• Repeat key messages using different methods;

• Provide better drug use alternatives.

REVIEW QUESTIONS

ESSAY QUESTIONS

1. Describe the concepts of essential drugs and rationale of drug use.
2. What are essential drugs and give some examples.
3. Explain briefly the rational use of drugs and add a short note on misuse and irrational use of drugs.
4. Discuss about the role of Pharmacist in rational use of drugs. Add a note on rational use of antibiotics.
5. Describe the chemotherapy of Urinary tract Infection and their rationale use.
6. Classify different types of Anaemia and indicate appropriate therapy with their rationale.

SHORT ANSWER QUESTIONS

7. Write a note on rational use of antibiotics.
8. Write a short note on misuse and irrational use of drugs.
9. What are essential drugs? Explain.
10. What is the role of Pharmacist in rational use of drugs?
11. Give the examples of non essential drugs.
    Enumerate the list of Essential drugs

BIBLIOGRAPHY / REFERENCES

1. Clinical Pharmacy and therapeutics by Roger Walker, Churchill Livingstone

2. Oxford American Handbook of Clinical Pharmacy by Michelle McCarthy and Denise R. Kockler

3. Basic Clinical Pharmacokinetics by Michael E. Winter, Lippincott Williams & Wilkins

4. Katzung, B.G.Basic and Clinical Pharmacology, Prentice hall, International.

5. Laurence, DR and Bennet PN. Clinical Pharmacology, Scientific book agency

6. Dr. D.R Krishna, V. Klotz, Clinical pharmaco kinetics, Springer Verlag

7. M Rowland and T N Tozer, "Clinical Pharmacokinetics" 2nd ed Lea & Fabiger, NY.

8. Lippincott Williams and Wilkins: Remington Pharmaceutical Sciences, 20th Edition.

9. Hamsten, Drug interaction, Kven Stockley.

10. Basic and clinical pharmacology- katzung, Mc Graw Hill

11. Grahame smith and Aronson, Clinical pharmacology and drug therapy

12. Richard A Helms, Text Book of Therapeutics Drug and Disease Management.

13. Herfindal E T and Hirschman JL, Williams and Wilkins, Clinical Pharmacy and therapeutics

14. Applied Therapeutics, The clinical uses of Drugs applied therapeutics INC

15. D. Abraham (Ed), Burger Medicinal chemistry ad Drug discovery, Vol. 1 & 2. John Wiley & Sons, New York 2003, 6ᵗʰ Ed.

16. Hospital Pharmacy - martin stevens